# THE FEEL-GOOD WAY

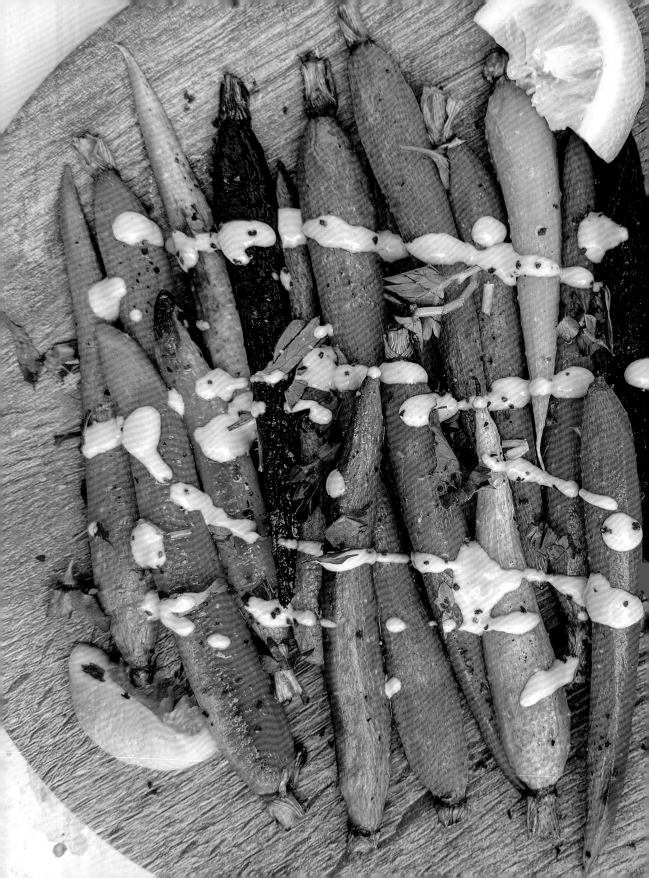

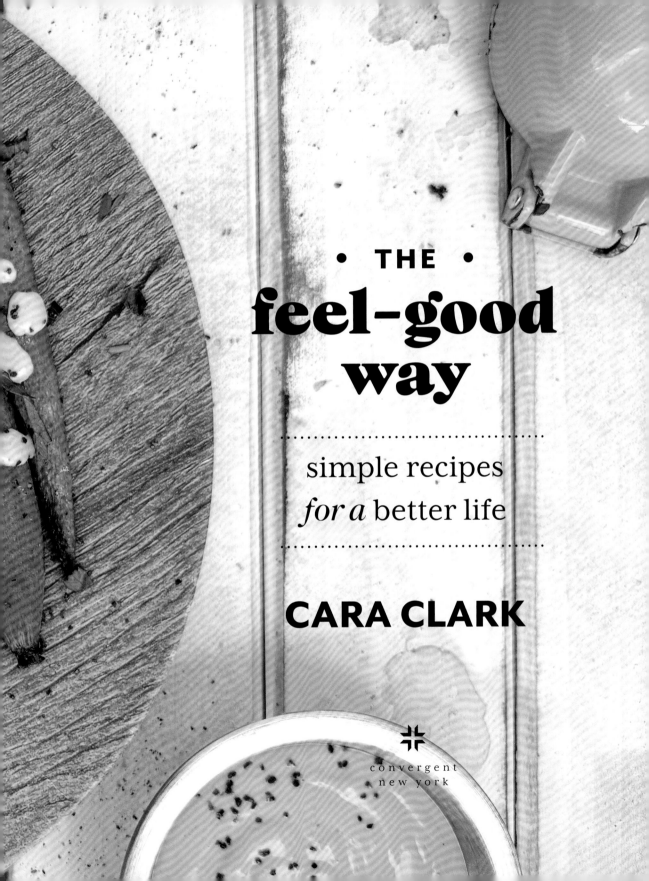

# THE
# feel-good
# way

simple recipes *for a* better life

## CARA CLARK

convergent
new york

Copyright © 2025 by Cara Clark
Foreword copyright © 2025 by Carrie Underwood
Lifestyle photographs by Angelica Zupanic copyright © 2025 by Angelica Marie Photography
Food photographs by Kim Cairns copyright © 2025 by Solstice Food Photography

Published in the United States by Convergent Books, an imprint of Random House, a division of Penguin Random House LLC, New York.

CONVERGENT BOOKS is a registered trademark and the Convergent colophon is a trademark of Penguin Random House LLC.

Library of Congress Cataloging-in-Publication Data
Names: Clark, Cara, author.
Title: The feel-good way / by Cara Clark.
Description: First edition. | New York, NY : Convergent, [2024] | Includes index.
Identifiers: LCCN 2024018086 (print) | LCCN 2024018087 (ebook) |
ISBN 9780593728048 (hardcover) | ISBN 9780593728055 (ebook) |
Subjects: LCSH: Cooking. | LCGFT: Cookbooks.
Classification: LCC TX714 .C52175 2024 (print) | LCC TX714 (ebook) |
DDC 641.5—dc23/eng/20240517
LC record available at https://lccn.loc.gov/2024018086
LC ebook record available at https://lccn.loc.gov/2024018087

Printed in China

convergentbooks.com

9 8 7 6 5 4 3 2 1

First Edition

Linen background by phatthanit/Adobe Stock;
bento box art by Stockhiu/Adobe Stock;
lunch box art by backup_studio/Adobe Stock

Book design by Elizabeth Rendfleisch

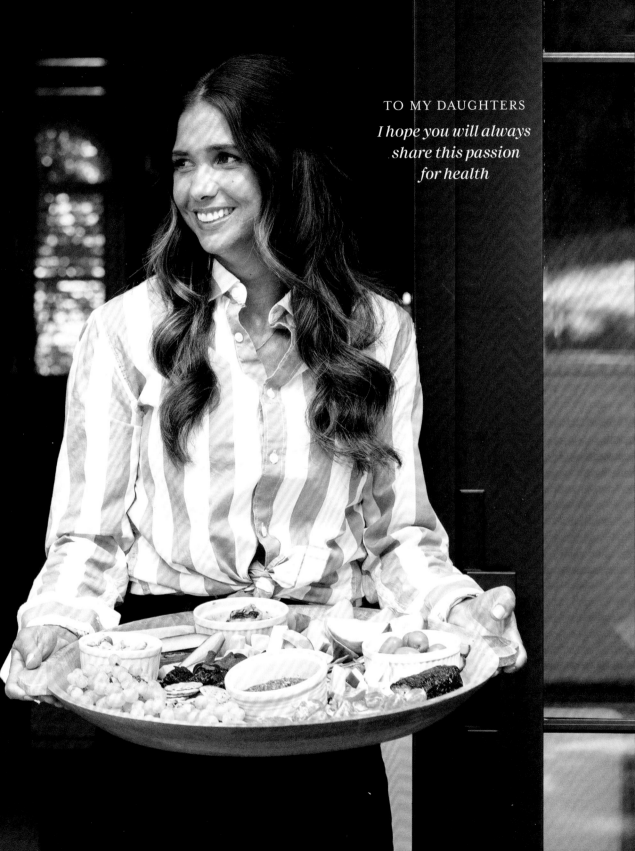

TO MY DAUGHTERS

*I hope you will always
share this passion
for health*

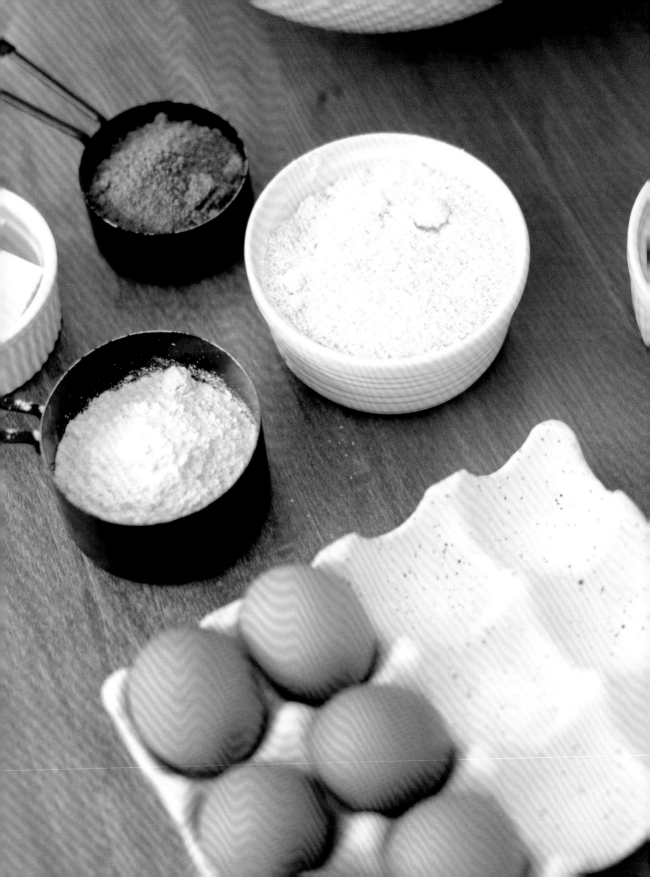

# FOREWORD

by carrie underwood

**Cara Clark has** always been someone whom I have greatly admired. I met her more than twenty years ago in a small classroom at Northeastern State University in Tahlequah, Oklahoma. Cara was a basketball player for the school, and I was a sorority girl who sang on the side. We ran in very different circles, but we shared many classes as we were both mass communication majors. Back then, I admired Cara's cool-girl style and her athleticism. Even though I have always considered myself semi-athletic (I grew up playing softball and even played a little basketball, thank you very much), I could not play like *that*. Plus, Cara seemed to be everyone's friend. She was gorgeous and kind. To be honest, it would've been quite difficult to find anyone who didn't like Cara.

After our time at NSU, we headed off on very different paths, but thankfully that would not be the end of our story. Flash forward a couple of decades, and it seems we were brought back into each other's lives through a bit of divine intervention. I'd love to say that "the Lord works in mysterious ways," but sometimes I think He's a little more obvious about the friendships He wants us to foster. Over the years, I had fallen in love with health and fitness. I had a demanding schedule full of travel and stress, and I realized that taking care of myself was the only way I could do my job at a level that reached my high personal expectations. I learned a lot, mainly through trial and error, and I decided to put what I had learned to good use and share it with others who might be looking to better their own health.

When I was writing my first book, *Find Your Path,* and developing my fitness app, fit52, a friend of mine brought to my attention that one of our former classmates was a dietitian and had a lot of great things going on in her life. Ahh, yes, I remembered Cara! So, I reached out and, just like that, the connection was reestablished. I sought her counsel on the nutrition side of things (after all, she was the expert), and before too long, Cara and her family even ended up moving east to my current hometown of Franklin, Tennessee.

These days, I still admire Cara, but for so many other reasons. Of course, that gorgeousness and athleticism has never gone away, but now I see her thriving as a wife, a mother to four beautiful, sweet young ladies, and an accomplished businesswoman. I see her juggling all the roles she has to play with kindness, love, and grace, and I see her taking care of herself and her family through all of it.

Cara's approach to diet and health is a lifestyle that is completely attainable for anyone who is seeking to take care of this one precious body God has given to them. Her way of life is not restrictive or gimmicky. Her simple, flavor-filled recipes are full of vitamins and nutrients from . . . wait for it . . . *real food*! This lifestyle is designed to make you feel good from the inside out. She believes we need to take care of our bodies, of course, but also our minds and our spirits. These things are all intertwined, and each deserves the same love and attention in order for us to feel good and live our best lives—for ourselves and for those we love.

I am blessed to continue to call Cara my friend and to have the opportunity to learn and grow from her expertise. By reading this book, now you can, too! Welcome to *The Feel-Good Way*.

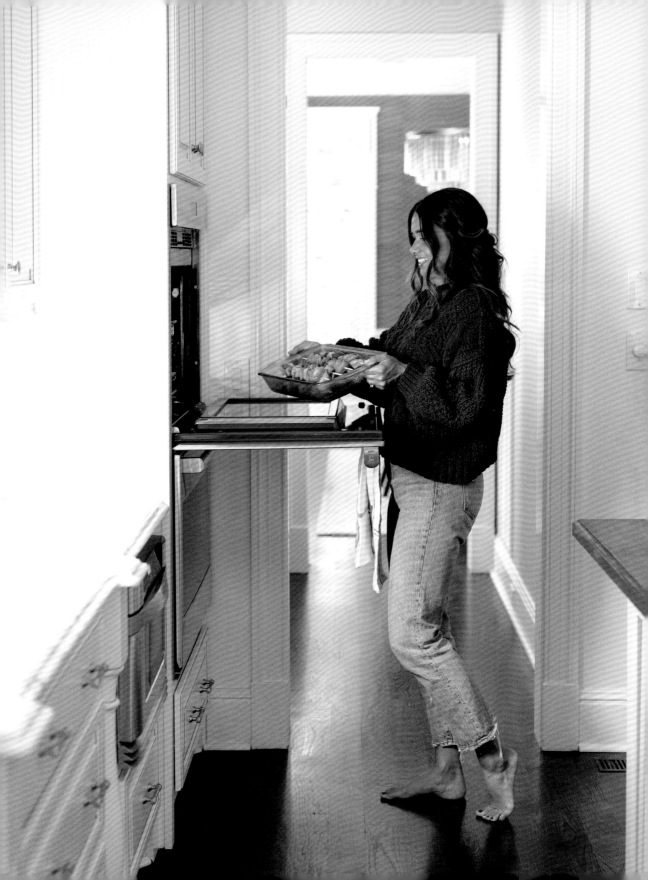

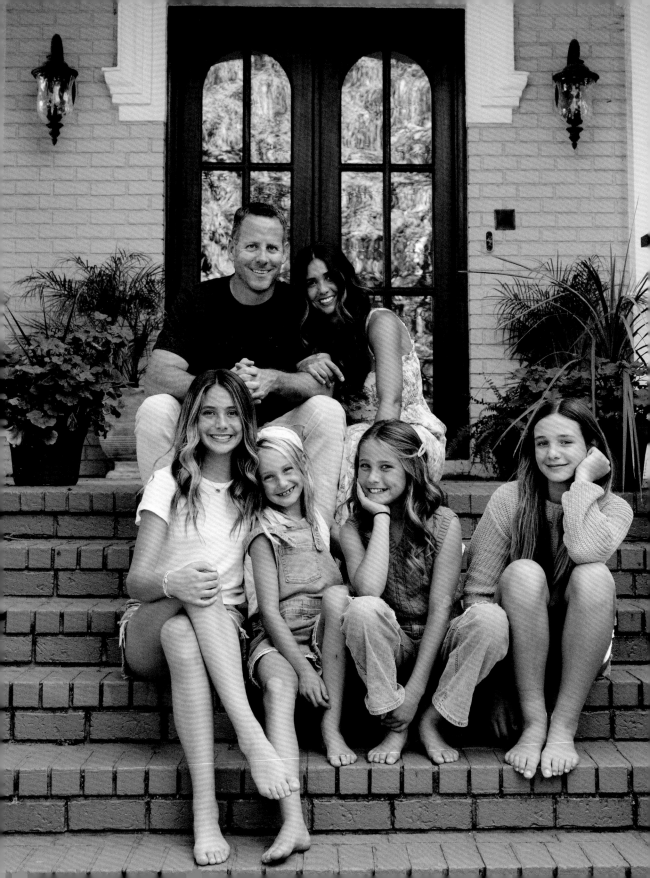

# CONTENTS

## Chapter 5  •  **DINNER** 178

## Chapter 6  •  **DESSERT** 220

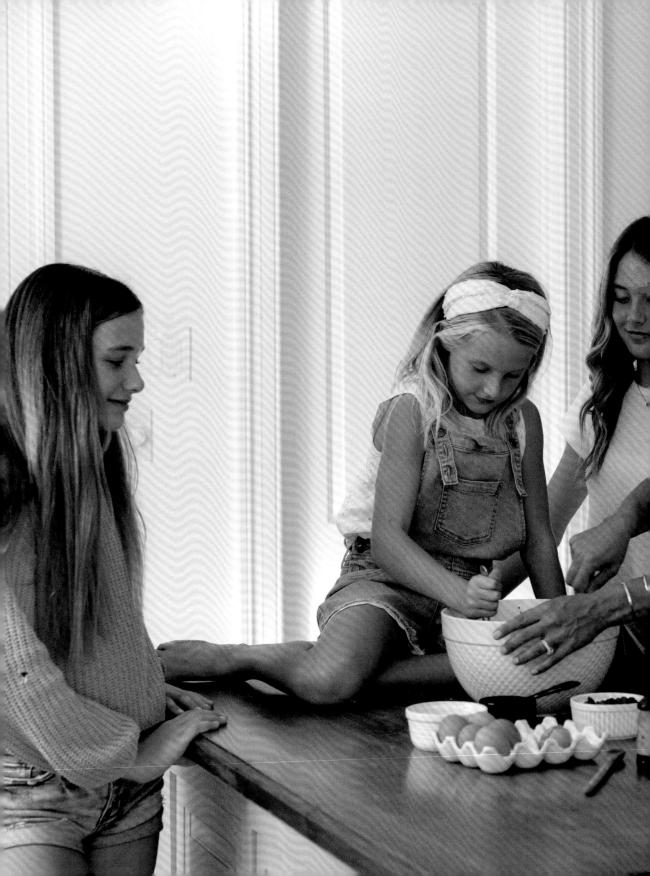

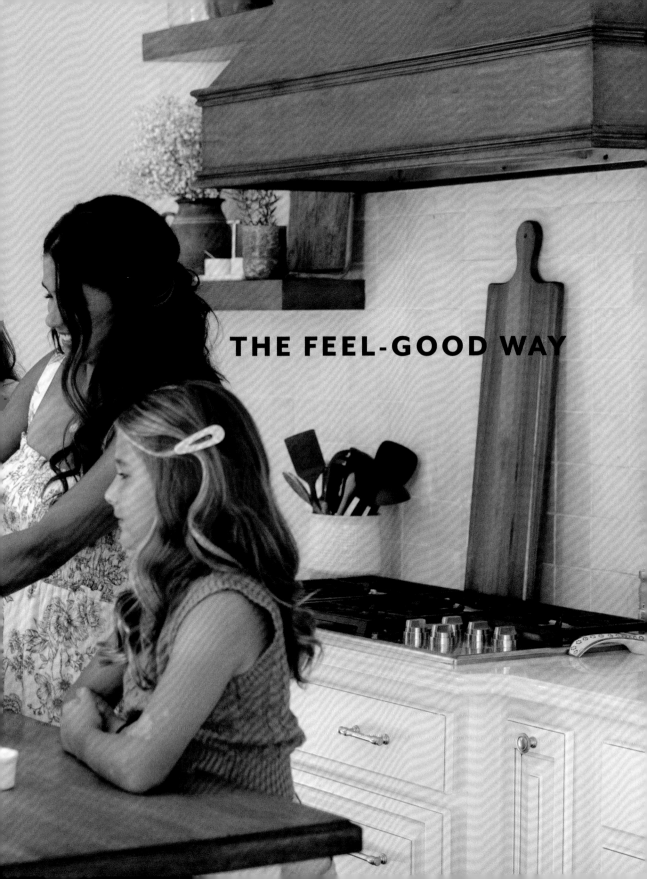

THE FEEL-GOOD WAY

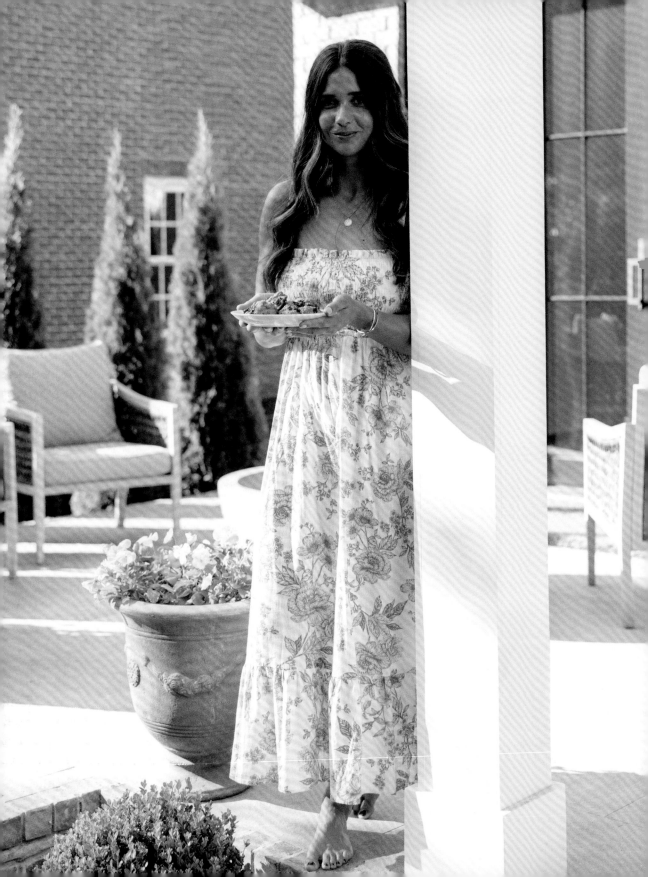

# WELCOME TO THE
# FEEL-GOOD WAY

*I'm Cara Clark.* I'm a certified sports and clinical nutritionist whose clients include celebrities, professional athletes, and regular people like you and me. I'm the mother of four girls and the wife of sixteen years to a picky eater. I played basketball in college. I'm an enneagram type two—the Caregiver. I love to cook and eat good food. And at the doctor's office, I'm one of those people who stand backward so I don't see my weight on the scale.

My health mission as the owner of Cara Clark Nutrition (CCN) is not about weight or calories or dieting. It's about feeling good emotionally and physically and helping others feel good without the pressure of trying to seek results on a scale. When I work with clients, I want them to look in the mirror and love and accept the person looking back at them. I want them to feel so good that they don't question the changes they're making or look forward to a date when they can go back to "normal." More than twenty thousand people have joined

me in my healthy eating challenges to date, and they tell me that because my philosophy isn't about numbers or restrictions, they feel free from cravings and binging. They say they have more energy and increased mental sharpness. And the added bonus is their clothes feel a little looser.

What does feeling good mean to me? It's having the energy to run around with my kids, seeing a glow in my skin and hair, thinking clearly without the fog, sleeping well, waking up refreshed, feeling comfortable in my clothes, and eating good food that's not a pain to prepare. It's teaching people to notice what food does to their bodies so they can trust themselves to eat the things they love without guilt, shame, or fear of gaining weight. And, for me, there's one more essential element to feeling good: a connection to God and my faith.

Ninety percent of my clients come to me looking for ways to improve not just their physical health but also their spiritual health. I started to understand this connection between physical and spiritual well-being better when I experienced it for myself. Around 2017, I became the sickest I've ever been, with mono-like symptoms, including exhaustion, sore throat, brain fog, insomnia, and nighttime anxiety. I met with integrative practitioners, including a functional medicine doctor, a doctor of Chinese medicine, and an acupuncturist. They put me on a healing protocol and encouraged me to lean in to my faith. As I began to feel better, I started to realize how much of my sickness was because of a neglect of my spiritual well-being. Even though I had been praying and was deeply rooted in my faith, I hadn't been tending to my spiritual self and the Holy Spirit living within me. Once I began to nourish my spirit with calming practices—listening prayer and meditation, cranial sacral therapy, infrared sauna sessions, and deep breathing—I started to understand the connection between spiritual health and the nervous system. It was a game changer for me.

As I started to work toward the improvement of my own holistic health, I better understood the cries for help that I'd been hearing from so many people who had reached out to me through emails,

DMs on social media, and in their personal assessments registering for my programs. I realized that the desperation of so many people who came to me went beyond their physical health to a neglect of their spiritual well-being. They were without hope. They felt like they had tried so many different programs and had failed. They didn't know where to turn next. People rarely came to me because they'd like to be a little healthier. Nine times out of ten, they came to me as a last-ditch effort. They were hopeless and defeated. I began to pivot my approach, understanding that my job was not only to give them hope by helping them feel better physically but also to recognize how their spiritual wounds and needs contributed to their struggle.

Physical and spiritual health are intertwined—it's hard to have one without the other, and they work the most beautifully when they work together, as I believe God intended. I've been on the same journey as so many of my clients, and I've personally experienced how getting in touch with your physical health and well-being can open up your connection to God. This connection is felt, not measured. When we feel good physically, it gives us energy to pursue a deeper state of wellness. Maybe

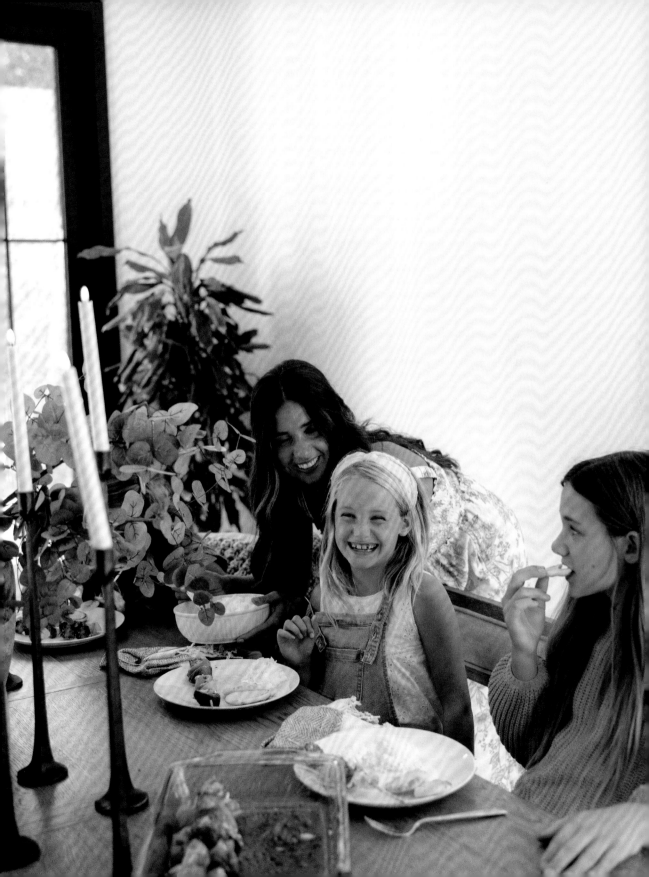

it comes through meditation or listening prayer. Maybe it's going for a walk or hike and smelling scents and hearing noises you've never noticed before because you haven't been connected to God's goodness and the beauty of nature.

Feeling good allows for a better sense of mindfulness of the world going on around us. For instance, if we feel poorly and we're driving in the car and someone cuts us off, our immediate reaction will likely reflect our state of being. If we feel good, we might be able to offer the person grace or even a wave or prayer in the moment. If we don't feel good, well . . . our reaction can be angry, overblown, and put us in a worse state than we were before. As we grow in our nutrition, we grow in our wellness and we grow in our potential to serve those around us with love and intention.

So, feeling good—inside and out—is what this book is all about. Wherever you are in your health and in your spirit right now—whether you're energized and hopeful or worn out and discouraged—let me welcome you to the *Feel-Good Way,* where just by starting to make the recipes, you are on your way to a sustainable lifestyle where your body and spirit can thrive like never before.

## BALANCING BLOOD SUGAR: THE SECRET TO FEELING BETTER

Do you ever feel like you want to crash at 2:00 P.M.? Are you addicted to that afternoon caffeine boost? Do you regularly crave something sweet and sugary in the afternoon? Something—anything—that will give you the energy to keep going? What's happening is an afternoon blood-sugar crash. When your blood sugar drops into hypoglycemic levels (too low), you are using energy from your muscles instead of from food, causing fatigue and lightheadedness. When you eat in a way that balances your blood sugar, you eliminate these hypoglycemic episodes that can lead to mood swings and cravings.

"Balancing blood sugar" sounds complicated, but it's pretty simple to follow the fundamentals that keep our blood sugar balanced on a cellular level. I will break it all down for you in more detail in the coming pages, but balancing blood sugar involves avoiding the glucose spike we get when we eat carbs on their own and instead slowing down the glucose by combining carbs with protein and fat when we eat. When you balance your blood sugar, you might notice the results almost instantly. The benefits

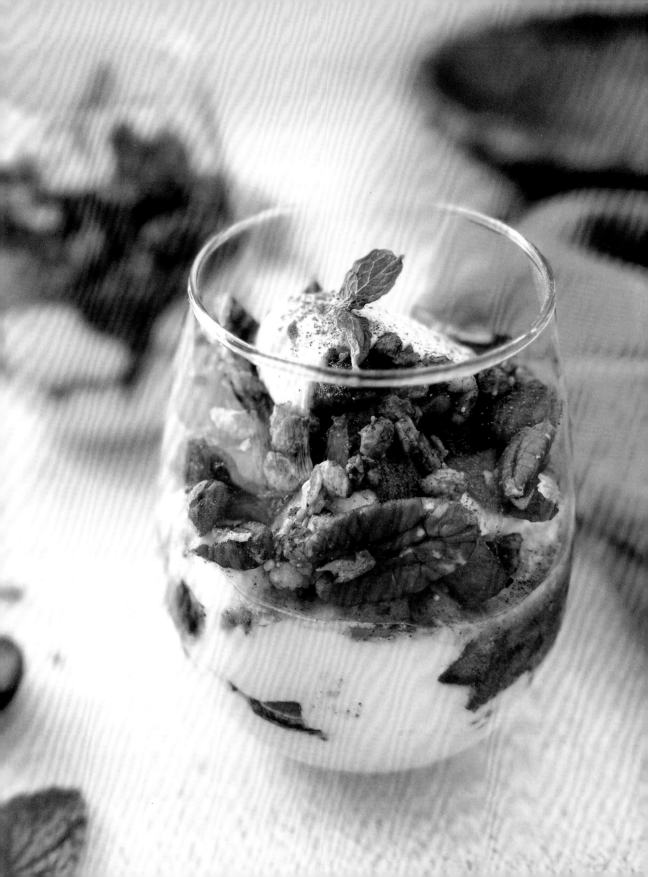

include having more energy, less brain fog, better moods, better sleep, stronger hair and nails, improved heart and gut health, and even the reversal of some autoimmune conditions—an overall improvement in quality of life. Once you understand this concept, it's hard to go back. You won't need that afternoon caffeine anymore! It's an easy lifestyle to adopt because, ultimately, you will feel better and be able to trust your hunger and fullness cues.

## COOKING AND EATING CAN FEEL GOOD

For many people who follow the Feel-Good fundamentals, weight loss is an added bonus, but my clients rarely mention pounds lost. Instead, they mention how much better they feel. This is not to say that our clients don't lose weight—they certainly do! But losing weight is no longer their primary focus once they actually feel good.

Our bodies are not calculators; therefore we should not be judged by calculations (goodbye, scale!). Results-driven, number-crunching diets have failed us over and over again, not just physically but mentally, too. I don't want my daughters growing up in a dieting culture. I'd like

them to be educated and confident in making purposeful food decisions. I don't want them to feel guilty for wanting a treat every now and then.

Life is meant to be lived and not overly controlled. When we control what we eat in a way that harms our metabolism or jeopardizes our immune system just so we can see the numbers go down on the scale, we are losing focus on what really matters. It's time to trust yourself, tap into your intuition, and live more fully. I will guide you on this journey through this book.

## FAITH IN FEELING BETTER

I've taught the foundation of food for more than fifteen years, but in the last seven or so, my clients have been asking for more. They want more than just information on their bodies and physical health. They want to understand the connection between physical wellness, mental health, and spiritual practices like listening prayer and meditation.

Take, for example, bloating—of all things! I have thousands of clients and members who have reduced their bloating just by setting their bodies into a restful state before eating. There are clinical and physical contributors to bloating, of course. But it's incredible what the body can do when it synchronizes with the nervous system. A prayer before meals, as well as breathing exercises, can reset the parasympathetic part of the nervous system, which does wonders for digestion.

As a person of faith, I firmly believe that God wants us well. He intricately designed our bodies in his likeness, and there is more going on inside us than meets the eye. Life is hard in countless uncontrollable ways. God calls on us to serve others, but when we are suffering, it's hard to serve. So many of my clients have gone through times of difficulty where just taking care of their families is all they can manage, and serving others or tending to their own needs is not feasible. But by making some changes, even small ones, you can feel better no matter what is happening in your life.

We are called to feel good, serve better, and live more fully in the moment. These are our goals in the *Feel-Good Way*. At the same time, health and emotional issues will inevitably arise, making it difficult to stay in the moment, especially if we don't have help to overcome them. That's where faith can come in and keep us afloat. Faith gives us hope on the deepest level. When we feel good physically, we are better able to commit to our faith—faith that will give

us the hope to sustain us through any circumstances.

Maybe you've suffered in the past and are still healing. Maybe you are suffering right now. We all experience suffering at some point and time. Taking care of yourself physically does not need to add to your hardship. Nor does it have to mean completely overhauling your life. It can start small—drinking more water, moving your body more or doing a different activity, eating even one meal a day from *The Feel-Good Way*. Any of these shifts can bring us closer to the healthiest version of ourselves. As we get healthier, our intuition gets stronger, and ultimately, so does our faith. Having a plan set in place that is good for our mind, body, and spirit—even if we're only doing a small part of it—helps us navigate the hard times with more surrender, peace, and hope.

Each day, I start by consecrating my work to God and praying about what he wants me to do. I pray over my client base and whatever projects are on my desk. And then I completely surrender the rest of my day to his will.

In this book, I share plenty of information about how what you eat relates to how you feel, including easy, delicious recipes. But I also include the daily prayers I make

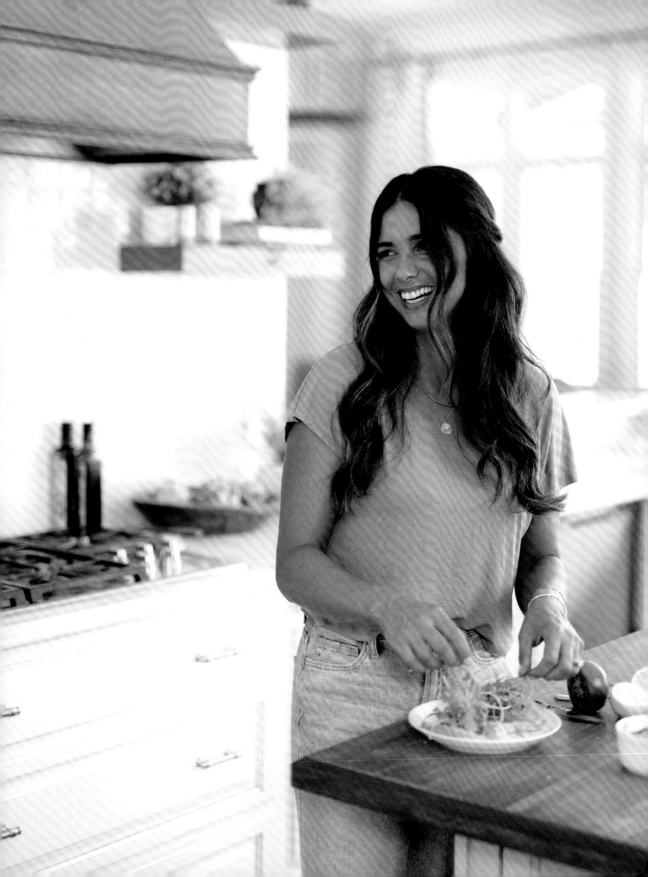

and the practices I do that help me stay connected to my ultimate purpose and well-being throughout each day. Feel free to skip these parts if you're not interested, but I share them in case they may help you start and stay on your journey to feeling better. I encourage you to explore the connection between your physical and spiritual health and feel for yourself how tending to both in harmony can work wonders in your life.

There's a lot to let go of when it comes to the kitchen. People come to me saying that they're busy, that they aren't good cooks, or that they hate cleaning up the mess. Because I grew up in a family of seven kids, things were always rush-rush in our kitchen. I've had to rewire my mindset that things can be calm in this space. My goal, both with these recipes and with the prayers and practices that accompany them, is to make you more

confident and help you show yourself more grace in this sacred space.

Real food takes some preparation, but I am thankful I have a family to clean up after, and thankful that I can support myself and my family with real food. As you adopt the Feel-Good lifestyle, I hope these mindset shifts will reflect in how you show up in this sacred space. You might find yourself having more kitchen dance parties or being more present when your kids share their biggest ideas, emotions, and dreams at the kitchen island while you do the dishes. You may find yourself getting chills during these moments of connection because you no longer resent your time and efforts in the kitchen.

As you begin this journey, my hope is that you're healing your body and spirit, leading not only to a Feel-Good Way but also to a Feel-Good Life. Let's get started!

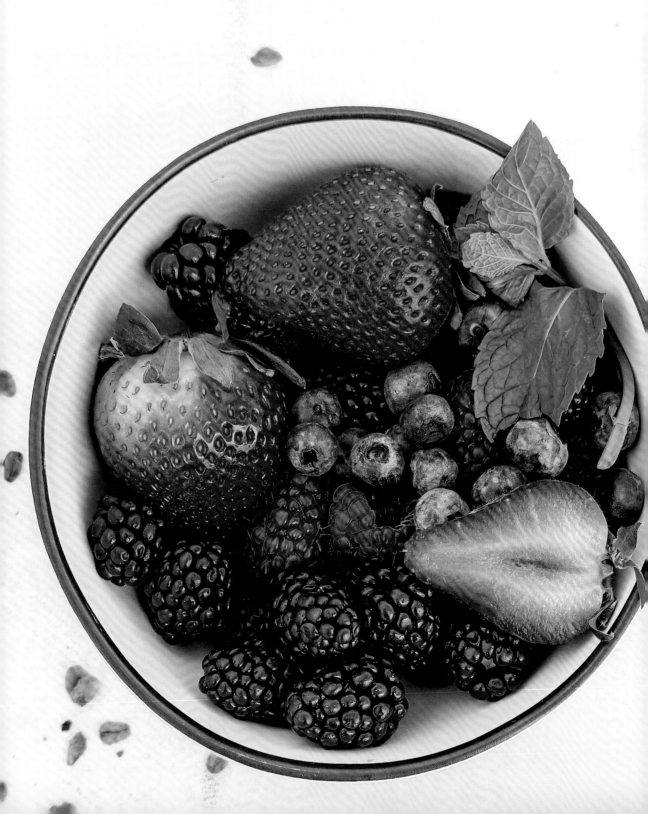

# FUNDAMENTALS

***My approach to*** eating is not all or nothing, and it doesn't like the word *no*. I'm not a big fan of rules, which can lead to guilt and giving up, but I do have some guidelines that help balance blood sugar and keep us mindful of what we're doing for our bodies and how it's affecting our level of energy.

These fundamentals are like building blocks. If you start doing even one of them, you will feel better. When you start to feel better, you start to feel hope, and that feeling of hope opens up all kinds of possibilities. These Feel-Good practices start when we wake up and then carry us through the day.

**1.** Combine macros—carbs, protein, and fat—every time you eat.

**2.** Eat within an hour of waking up, then eat a meal or snack every four hours.

**3.** Eat the rainbow! Try to eat five different colors every day.

**4.** Drink at least eighty ounces of water every day.

**5.** Move your body at least four times a week for at least thirty minutes, doing an activity that feels good to you.

You may not get as excited as I do about the science behind these fundamentals, but in my experience, when I feel like I understand *why* I am doing something and *how* it's functioning, I'm more committed to making it happen. So let me offer some information on how these fundamentals work within our bodies to make us feel better.

## 1. COMBINE MACROS—CARBS, PROTEIN, AND FAT—EVERY TIME YOU EAT

Macronutrients, or "macros," are carbs, protein, and fat. Our bodies need all three of these to function well. The best balance for most people's diets would be to have around 50 percent carbs, 20 percent protein, and 30 percent fat in each meal. I often see people undereating in hopes that it will help them achieve a body mass they're happy with. If they indulge in a Starbucks latte, for example, they won't eat lunch in order to offset their calories for the day. Or they might grab a piece of fruit to compensate for their choice. Both the latte and the fruit are mostly carbs, though, and eating them causes a spike in blood sugar, a sugar rush leading to excess fat storage and likely more cravings throughout the rest of the day.

On the opposite end, I've seen clients try to offset a choice of, say, a burger by not eating the bun or any carbs with it. Many people come to me feeling low in energy and "in a fog," and a lot of the time, these symptoms are directly related to the fact that they aren't eating *enough* carbs.

The long game here is that as you learn to eat to regulate your blood sugar, not only will you feel better but you will also reduce the guilt you feel making food choices. You'll learn how to enjoy the latte but maybe add egg bites and a small fruit on the side. You'll appreciate the chance to indulge in a delicious burger with a bun—carbs and all.

We need carbs for glucose, which is what gives us energy. That being said, not all carbs are created equal. Natural, complex, high-fiber carbs are best—meaning fruits and vegetables, whole grains, and beans. Simple carbs, such as sweets, processed foods with added sugar or sugar substitutes, cookies and crackers, soda, chips, and so on, do not give us the same benefits as complex carbs.

Protein, the second macro, is foundational to the development and upkeep of healthy muscles, blood, hair, nails, skin, hearts, and brains. It's essential for creating enzymes, which help speed up chemical

# macros 101

**protein**

wild fish, shrimp/shellfish, canned tuna, sashimi sushi

chicken breast, turkey breast, lean ground turkey breast, ground chicken breast

bison, venison, grass-fed beef sirloin and tenderloin, very lean grass-fed ground beef

nutritional yeast, egg whites

collagen peptides, protein powder

**fats + protein**

ground turkey, bacon, steak, bone-in skin-on meats, duck, grass-fed ground beef, jerky/chomps sticks, wild salmon/ fatty fish, whole eggs, nuts/nut butters, seeds/seed butters, hummus, cheese

**fats**

olive oil, avocado oil, coconut oil, sesame oil

grass-fed butter, ghee

avocado or coconut oil mayo, egg yolks, avocados

**all three macros**

avocados,* peanuts, beans and legumes, CCN smoothies, CCN meals, pizza, protein bars, sandwiches/wraps, 2% or full-fat plain Greek yogurt,** 2% or full-fat cottage cheese**

**protein + carbs**

oats/oatmeal, quinoa, chickpea pasta, whole grain pasta, wild rice, sprouted grains, amaranth, buckwheat, peas

**fats + carbs**

olives, fried foods, chocolate, ice cream, coconut milk, unsweetened coconut flakes, coconut yogurt (a lot of hyper-satiating processed foods)

**carbs**

fruits, dried fruit

breads, tortillas, cereals

most granolas

potatoes, rice

honey, maple syrup, coconut sugar

winter squash, pumpkin

corn

root veggies

non-starchy vegetables***

*mostly fat
**mostly fat and protein
***colorful non-starchy veggies contain carbs (however, the total grams are quite low), and some contain some protein—consider these an unlimited food

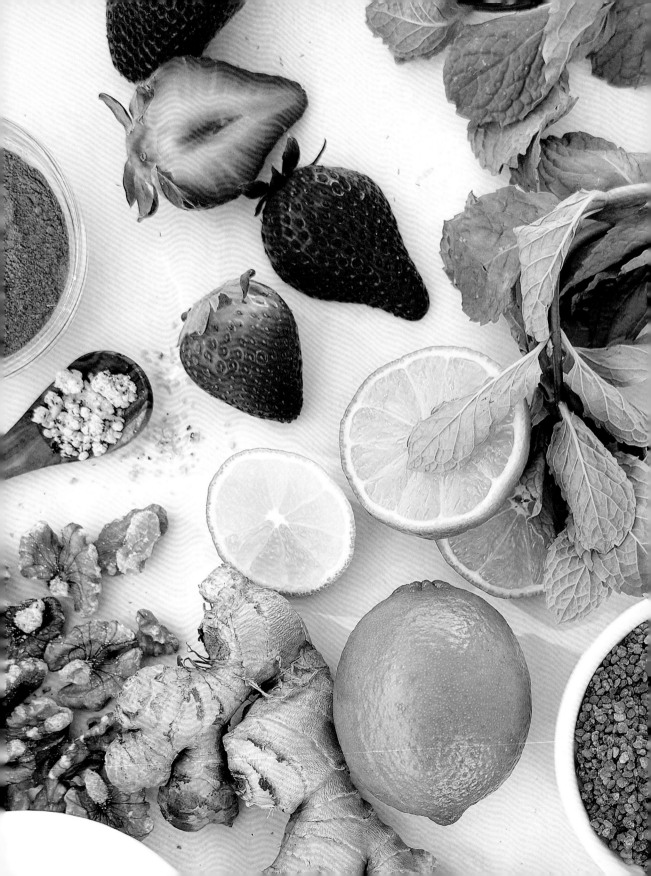

reactions in our body—particularly our livers and digestive tracts. Protein is also the building block for most of the hormones secreted by the pituitary gland. That's a lot of jobs—but when you're not eating enough carbs and fat, protein has to step in as the primary energy source, and there won't be enough protein left over to do its essential work developing and maintaining healthy organs and systems in the body.

These days, people really lean in to protein, thinking it's the primary source of everything. But as with many things in life, too much of a good thing isn't a good thing. Each macronutrient has essential roles, but not one is more important than the others. My recommended protein sources are lean meats and wild-caught seafood, eggs, beans, nuts and seeds, organic dairy, and quinoa.

Fat, the third macro, provides our body with its most concentrated form of energy. It also slows digestion, helping us feel full longer. Fat aids the absorption of vitamins, and it's essential for creating biochemicals like hormones and antibodies and for the health of our circulatory, immune, lymph, and nervous systems. It even contributes to healthy cell membranes, which leads to more hydrated and "plumped-up" skin.

All to say, it's time to let go of the asso-ciation between body fat and healthy dietary fat. By allowing appropriate amounts of healthy fats into your diet, you are supporting your body, not making it fatter. Healthy fat sources include dairy, eggs, lean meats, wild-caught seafood, healthy oils, ghee, grass-fed butter, avocados, and nuts and seeds.

You may notice that some foods—like nuts, yogurt, legumes, and even some grains—contain more than one macro. Quinoa, whole grains such as rice and oats, and legumes such as black beans and chickpeas do, too. If you're eating these foods, you can count them as multiple macros at once.

### HOW THIS MAKES US FEEL GOOD

So, why do we combine these three macros every time we eat? The short answer: This combination causes us to burn fat all day, feel fuller, and have more energy and healthy brain function. Our body loves these three macros together. Eating them in combination is how we feel good and ensure that our body is working as it should.

The longer, more scientific answer is this: This combination of macros when we eat helps us manage our blood sugar. Carbohydrates are converted to glucose when they hit our bloodstream. When eaten *alone*, though, carbs spike our blood glucose, creating a quick need to get rid of the excess right away. When there is excess glucose, it stores first as glycogen in the liver and muscles and then in our adipose tissue as fatty acid for when it's needed. When we eat excess carbohydrates and not enough fat or protein, we feel a burst of energy, but then it quickly drops because all the excess energy is being stored away.

However, when we *combine* the three macronutrients and energy sources each time we eat, we provide our bodies with sustainable and usable energy. We get a slow rise of glucose, instead of a quick burst. This slow release gives the energy-transfer process time to use the appropriate amount of energy. During this process, our bodies use stored fat for output. When we use stored fat for energy, we feel balanced, stable, and *good*. Our brain becomes clearer and sharper, and our liver can do its job better as well. We can feel the difference in the sustainable release of energy and also in the way we look and the way our clothes fit.

Our macronutrients need each other to function best. We feel good when our bodies are functioning optimally and utilizing energy from food. You'll notice in the upcoming recipes that the meals are already macro balanced. If they're not, we indicate what to add on the side to balance them. To give you a general idea of a meal that's macro balanced, imagine on a plate a 4-ounce chicken breast and 1 cup of starchy carbs like a grain or root vegetable, topped with a healthy oil or ghee and a colorful non-starchy vegetable. It's that simple!

## 2. EAT WITHIN AN HOUR OF WAKING UP, THEN EAT A MEAL OR SNACK EVERY FOUR HOURS

Instead of restricting calories, eat small meals or snacks on a consistent basis throughout the day. When you eat this way, it fuels your body so it can function as it should, including burning fat and stabilizing blood sugar.

### HOW THIS MAKES US FEEL GOOD
When we don't eat enough calories, we may lose weight in pounds, but it's usually a loss of muscle tissue instead of fat. When we eat regularly and combine our macros, we allow our body to burn stored fat from places like our belly, thighs, and butt. Eating healthy snacks throughout the day helps us maintain a steady blood sugar, which allows our bodies to function

optimally rather than being stressed or deprived. When our bodies are functioning as they should, we have increased metabolism and energy and are able to burn fat and gain muscle.

When we don't fuel our body properly all day long, our body feels deprived. It cries out for nutrients via headaches, cravings, low energy, grumpiness, and all manner of health problems. Answer the call. Eat! And when you feel full, stop eating.

Hunger and fullness cues will become more obvious once you've been following our food philosophy for a couple of weeks. You just have to start trusting yourself. To really tap into your fullness cues, slow down your eating and try to get more chews on every bite. When you eat small meals throughout the day, you will feel less hungry because you are giving your body what it needs to fuel itself. The size of your meals may be smaller than when you ate only two or three meals a day, but you will feel much better after eating.

## 3. EAT THE RAINBOW! TRY TO EAT FIVE DIFFERENT COLORS EVERY DAY

No, I'm not talking about multicolored "fruity"-flavored cereals. I mean eating five different colors put there by Mother Nature and not additives. Colors to eat in your rainbow include green (asparagus and kiwi); blue and purple (blueberries and red cabbage); yellow (squash and peaches); orange (carrots and tangerines); white (bananas and cauliflower); brown (mushrooms and ginger); and red (bell peppers and watermelon). One of the easiest ways to get in more colors is to make a delicious smoothie.

### HOW THIS MAKES US FEEL GOOD
Fruits and vegetables get their colors from phytochemicals: compounds produced by plants that help them resist infections from pathogens, such as fungi, bacteria, and viruses. In fact, treatments for viral diseases are beginning to incorporate more plant-based products, because the phytochemicals from plants cause fewer side effects, are less toxic, and don't increase resistance.

Each phytochemical from each plant has its own unique benefit to the body; the greater variety of fruits and vegetables you eat, the more distinct benefits you will get. Red fruits and veggies have compounds and nutrients known to be cancer fighters, antioxidants, and inflammation reducers. They're good for your memory, your lungs, your heart, blood pressure, and cholesterol.

Orange and yellow fruits and veggies benefit your eyes, skin, hair, and joints. They can also boost immunity, fight cell-damaging free radicals, and build healthy bones and teeth.

Green fruits and veggies reduce the risk of certain cancers, promote heart health, ease digestion, support healthy vision, boost the immune system, and cut down cell-damaging free radicals.

Blue and purple fruits and veggies are antiaging, and they support brain, heart, digestive, and eye health. They also can boost immunity, lower cholesterol, improve calcium absorption, and act as powerful cancer fighters by reducing free radicals and fighting inflammation and tumor growth.

Brown and white fruits and veggies possess antiviral, antifungal, and antibacterial properties. They serve as powerful immune boosters, hormone balancers, and cancer fighters, helping reduce the risk of colon, breast, and prostate cancers.

So, why limit yourself? Eat the rainbow and get the whole shebang of benefits. Not sure how to work all the colors into your meals? That's what this cookbook is all about. Check out the recipes and get busy in your Feel-Good kitchen.

## 4. DRINK AT LEAST 80 OUNCES OF WATER EVERY DAY

This simply means drinking the good stuff we are so blessed to have access to all day long. If you get a 40-ounce water bottle and fill it up once in the morning and once in the afternoon, it's easy to keep track of your intake, so make sure you've always got it right there with you.

### HOW THIS MAKES US FEEL GOOD

Water comprises 75 percent of our bodies! We need it constantly to transport nutrients to cells, remove waste products from the body, and basically keep everything working and moving inside our bodies in a balanced and effective way. Sometimes when we feel hungry or cranky or have a headache, what we're really suffering from is dehydration. Feel better quickly with more water!

## 5. MOVE YOUR BODY AT LEAST FOUR TIMES A WEEK FOR AT LEAST THIRTY MINUTES, DOING AN ACTIVITY THAT FEELS GOOD TO YOU

This means physical activity that raises your heart rate for thirty minutes. If you have

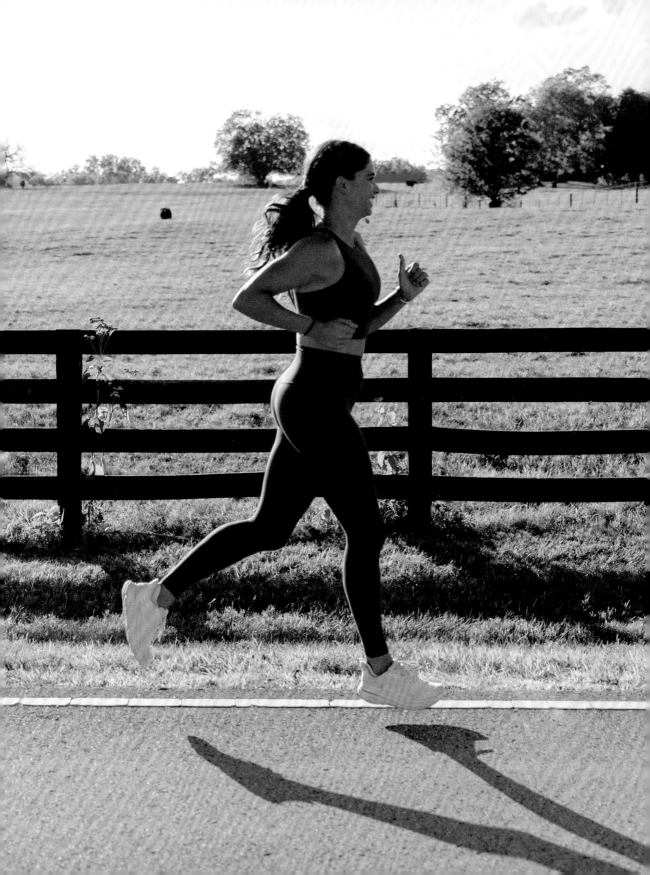

no preexisting health conditions, you may want to get into your target heart rate. You can calculate that by taking 220, subtracting your age, and trying to hit 65 to 85 percent of that rate. For example, I'm forty years old, so my target heart rate is between 117 and 153. This is the rate where I'm burning fat for energy. If I'm above that rate, I'll be tapping into glycogen storage and burning sugar for immediate energy instead of fat cells that will give me more sustainable energy throughout the day. If I'm below my target rate, I'm not quite burning enough to get my body working.

Avoid overexercising and pushing yourself to exhaustion. If you feel exhausted from your workouts, it's too much or not the right workout. We should feel happy, energized, strong, and healthy after our workouts.

**HOW THIS MAKES US FEEL GOOD**
Exercise helps boost our mental and emotional states more than any drug or self-help program on the market. As long as you maintain the target heart rate for thirty minutes, you'll be very efficiently burning fat as your fuel source and you'll feel energized afterward. When we overexercise, we start depleting muscle instead of fat, increase inflammation in our joints, and put wear on our bodies. Afterward we might feel nauseous, achy, and super fatigued when we should be feeling energized and empowered.

# FEEL-GOOD FAQ

. . . . . . . . . . . . . . . . . . . . . . . . . . . . . . . . . . . . . . . . . . . . . . . . . . .

**It's been so long since I've worked out regularly, and the idea of getting back into a fitness routine is overwhelming. Where do I start?**

Not everyone is born with a natural desire to run bleachers or do push-ups with a smile on their face. If you *are* one of those people, good for you! But for everybody else, exercise can feel like one more thing to cross off your list. We know we need exercise, but we may dread it or feel like we don't have the energy for it. I hear this from clients a lot.

If this sounds like you, walking is likely the best place for you to start. Walking is gentle on our musculoskeletal system, as well as our adrenal system. Here's the bottom line: As we build our health, we need to be intuitive with our movement the way we are with our food. As we venture into new territory, moving our bodies can feel like one more thing to do, but walking is an innate activity that should be part of our every day. It benefits our body and spirit.

Keep in mind that it may not be the intimidation factor or you not having a natural-born passion for working out that's contributing to your lack of motivation to get started. It's likely that your attitude toward exercising is influenced by the depletion of hormones when you exercise, especially if you're not eating in a way that nourishes your hormonal balance. So, how can you feel more motivated to exercise? I will give you a line that you will see me repeat in one form or another many times: It starts with food.

If you start to eat according to the Feel-Good Way fundamentals, using the recipes in this book, you are kicking off a long list of positive benefits, including eating regularly, which contributes to balancing your cortisol (stress hormone) and melatonin (sleep hormone). When you sleep at night, having nourished your body well all day rather than with food that makes you feel unwell, you get a better, deeper sleep, giving you more energy the next day. When you have more energy, you feel more motivated to exercise. When you begin to exercise, you burn energy in a positive way so that at night you're appropriately tired, then you get good sleep, and on the cycle goes.

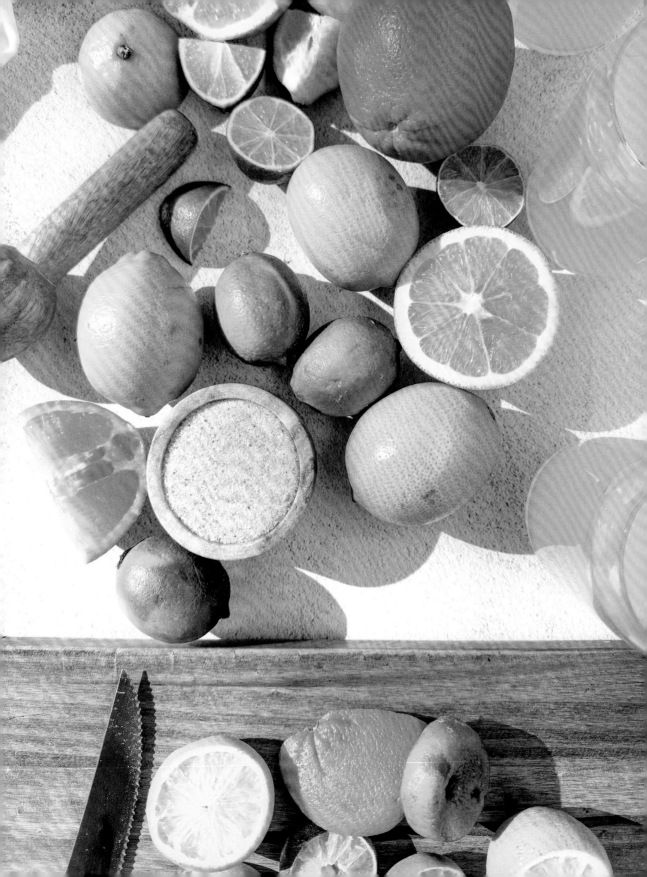

Better food in your body equals better sleep, leading to more energy and desire to exercise, which creates even more energy and even better sleep. It's all connected, and it all starts with putting food in your body that nourishes rather than depletes. As you begin to incorporate exercise into your life, you'll notice you actually feel better moving your body when it's being supported by the good food you've been giving it, and it can release hormones that improve your mood and your mind.

As you begin, start with an activity you enjoy. Maybe that's yoga, Pilates, or a long walk in the hills (my personal favorite!). Maybe it's pickleball or simply walking your dog. Whatever you choose, do it in the same way I'm encouraging you to choose your food: If it feels good, your body is loving it. If it feels bad, leaves you fatigued, depletes your daily energy, or causes injury, it's not the right exercise for your current stage of life. Your body gives you warnings when something isn't working for it, so it's important to pay attention. If you feel a little tired, try adding some electrolytes—such as coconut water, a granule of Celtic sea salt, or even a premade mix—before, during, or after exercise. If you immediately feel better, that could be your answer. But if you consistently feel bad or have headaches from exercise, you might need to slow down or completely switch it up. Exercise should enhance your health, not deplete it.

When you get to that sweet spot of finding the right level of exercise intensity, the hormones being released will lift your mood and connect your spirit to your mind and body. There is magic behind movement and exercise that goes so far beyond burning calories or giving us "results." Find your Feel-Good level of movement and savor the sensation.

## HOMEMADE ELECTROLYTE DRINK

**MAKES 1 DRINK**

Juice of ½ orange

Juice of ½ lemon

Juice of 1 lime

¼ teaspoon Celtic or other sea salt

12 ounces water

Ice as needed

Combine ingredients in your favorite glass, jar, or water bottle and enjoy!

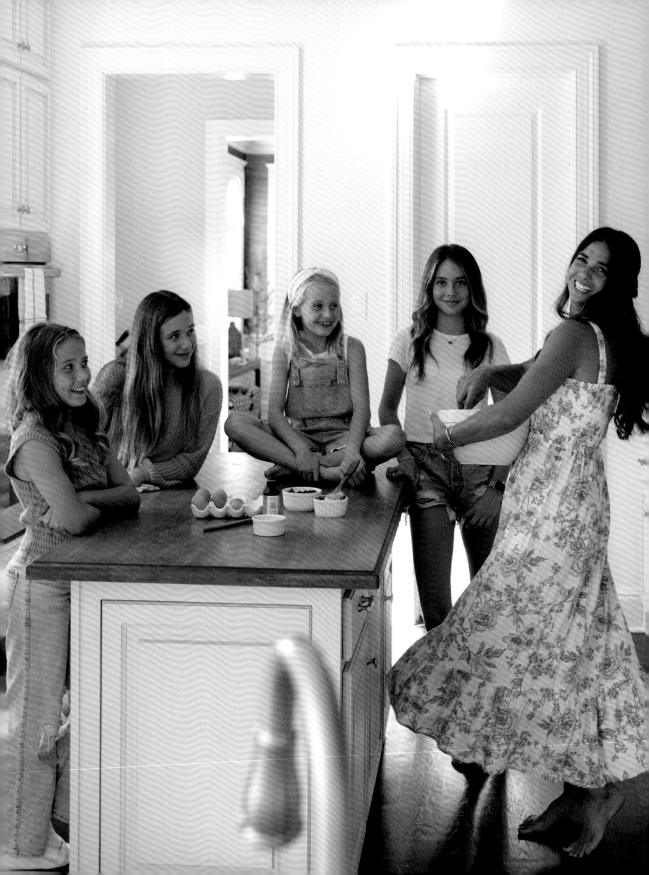

# FUELED BY
# FOOD AND FAITH

························································

## *the feel-good mindset*

**This book is** organized to help you connect with yourself, your body, and your spirit all the way from sunup, through lunch and the busy afternoon, and finally to family time and winding down. There are recipes for breakfast; for smoothies, shakes, and bowls; for lunch; for snacks; for dinner; and for dessert. In each chapter, I'll not only provide recipes, but also give you some helpful information, nutritional education, prayers, and inspiration to keep you fueled, body and soul. You don't need to eat six full meals a day, so you might not reference every chapter every single day. But every recipe in this book can serve as any meal, so you might find that you enjoy making a dessert for lunch or a smoothie for dinner. All the recipes are consistent in size, so feel free to mix them up to suit your needs and lifestyle.

Be your own guide. You are learning how to be the expert on your body. Trust how you feel. The numbers lie, but how you feel does not. Rewiring your mind and spirit to understand that *you* know best has its challenges, but once you accept that you're the boss and you get to create your own path with the tools we're suggesting, you are so much more likely to succeed.

As I've mentioned, if you do nothing other than start making and eating the recipes in this book, you will feel better! To take the Feel-Good Way to the next level, here are some concepts to keep in mind that I've learned through science and personal experience.

## INTUITIVE EATING

Eating nutrient-rich foods that nourish rather than deprive the body is the only way to maintain a healthy lifestyle long-term. The recipes in this book are a great place to start. Try the recipes, listen to how your body responds, and welcome yourself to the "diet" that could never be a fad: intuitive eating.

What I mean by *intuitive eating* is becoming the expert on your own body. Counting calories, restricting your eating, even losing weight—none of this matters if you don't tune in to the signals your body is sending at any given moment. Only you know what feels healthy and right in your own body and mind.

So many things can shift our energy needs, such as exercise, menstruation, stress, general activity level, and more. Not only that, but food intolerance can also pop up during times of stress or different cycles of the month or even during a full-on hormone/life transition. For me, I'm totally fine with organic corn and products of organic corn until around my menstrual cycle, when corn can be inflammatory for me. Understanding our bodies and the changing needs can only come from intuitive understanding and mindfulness.

When you feel hungry, eat! Turn to real foods that come from nature—fruits, veggies, whole grains, beans, nuts, lean meats, and dairy. Or make a recipe from any chapter of this book. We live in the moment,

right? We should eat in the moment, too, and appreciate the nourishment healthy food gives to our bodies.

As you eat, chew slowly and enjoy every bite. Eating slowly gives time for leptin—the hormone that tells you when you feel full—to be released and make its way from the stomach to your brain. Listen to your body and recognize when you feel full. It's easy to say, "Eat when you're hungry, then stop when you're full." In real life, I know it's not always that simple. When you've had a history of dieting or an unhealthy relationship with food (I'm speaking from personal experience here!), it can be a serious challenge to stop, listen to ourselves and our bodies, and trust what they are telling us. Start with nutrient-rich foods—they are your friend in every way—and you will be giving your body and mind the fuel they need to work together to send and receive the right signals of hunger and satiation.

Another way we can be more intuitive about our eating is recognizing when we're emotionally hungry rather than physically hungry. We all know what it's like to eat in response to stress, nerves, guilt, depression, and the countless other emotions that strike us during the day. When this emotional pull occurs, pay attention to it. Do you feel a pit in your stomach that could only be comforted by food? Do you feel a nervous energy that is driving what you're hungry for? Do you need a pleasure response to take the edge off? Acknowledge what you're feeling, then instead of rushing to consume unhealthy food—which will not make you feel better—try to find another outlet. Fix yourself a cup of herbal tea, go for a walk, exercise, play with your child or pet, take a bubble bath, listen to music, journal, or call a friend. Any of these alternatives will leave you feeling better, unlike turning to unhealthy food.

Intuitive eating is a learned habit. As you develop your intuition, you will feel more nourished and energized and less restricted. There will be times when you want to eat more than the suggested serving amount and times when you want less. Let your intuition be your ultimate guide so you can truly understand the difference.

As you're learning to listen to yourself and developing your intuition, give yourself grace and patience. Intuitive eating takes practice! And none of us is perfect. We all make mistakes on our daily path to feeling good. Feeling guilty about our missteps only makes it worse. So, accept that you won't always make the best choices and remind yourself why you're on this journey in the first place: to feel better.

## MOVING AWAY FROM AN ALL-OR-NOTHING MENTALITY

Related to the fact that we are not perfect, the misstep I see most often with clients and friends is the idea that when it comes to our eating lifestyle, it's either all or nothing. Too many of us feel like either we have to be a strict vegan who does yoga, runs marathons, and never eats sweets, or there's no point—so we might as well just eat an excess of junk food and not bother exercising. Forget the extremes. There is a happy medium! Feeling good is not an all-or-nothing enterprise.

First of all, what you eat has no inherent morality. Food is not good or bad, and you are not a bad person when you eat something that doesn't qualify as healthy. Second, if you do eat something you wish you hadn't, then you don't have to throw in the towel and eat in an unhealthy way the rest of the day or the week. Move on with the mindset of a new start and a new beginning. Remind yourself, *I eat healthy because it makes me happy and makes me feel good. I love feeling good! Eating right lets me enjoy my life and live it to the fullest.*

One way to keep from getting stuck in the all-or-nothing trap is to avoid restricting yourself too much from the start. If

# FEEL-GOOD FAQ

## Should I weigh myself or not?

I get this question a lot. If you have been on and off different diet programs in the past that didn't result in a long-term healthy lifestyle, it may be hard to try a new philosophy without a weight-loss goal in mind. Some people use a scale chronically as a means to measure success. Others never weigh themselves except when required at doctor appointments or wellness exams. Weight can be such an emotional trigger. The number on the scale doesn't paint a very complex picture, yet our bodies are so beautifully complex. A negative result on the scale can send us into depression or cause us to overexercise and deplete our bodies of needed nutrition. A positive result can lead us to out-of-control indulgence. Either result may be fleeting, but we may act on it as if it's written in stone. Weight is never a measure of our worth, yet it can change the way we see ourselves.

Personally, I am not a fan of scales, for all the reasons we've already discussed, but weighing yourself is totally up to you. If you need the data for the purpose of recognizing progress, I get that. I still recommend logging how you *feel* each day so you can start to associate progress more with feeling rather than the number on the scale. And if you do weigh yourself, I would suggest not getting on the scale more than once a week. I've worked with so many people who have overused the scale to the point that they can't even reflect on how they feel relative to the food they're eating. If you can't get away from the number and you can't step back and consider how you're feeling in your body, then the number is meaningless anyway. What does a number mean when it doesn't translate to feeling good?

We don't want our weight to be more important than how we're feeling. Typically, how we feel is what sustains us while the weight falls into place.

you've decided to completely eliminate a food from your diet or label something as "off-limits," chances are you're going to obsess about it and even crave it. Allow yourself a treat every now and then. Plan it out in advance and don't feel bad for looking forward to it. Instead of an all-or-nothing approach, shoot for eating well 80 to 90 percent of the time and indulging 10 to 20 percent of the time. The 80/20 rule is what I like to call living life.

## DEVELOPING CONFIDENCE IN THE KITCHEN AS AN ACT OF SERVICE AND LOVE

The greatest gift I have on this earth is my family. Having four daughters, all eager to learn how to operate a kitchen themselves, I want to be confident and show them how cooking and eating is a positive and fun experience. Being confident in the kitchen is not about becoming the best fine-dining cook—it's about providing a nutritious meal that supports your family's needs. Confidence comes from knowing you have the tools, literal and figurative, to do this. As my team and I have worked with thousands of families over the years, some of my favorite feedback is when people say they have become more confident in their

cooking—that they're actually enjoying the kitchen for the first time in their lives.

If you haven't been confident cooking in the past and are feeling hesitant about learning a bunch of new methods and ingredients, don't worry! These recipes are simple and straightforward, with step-by-step instructions. How nice will it be to feel good about what you're eating as you're gaining confidence in a new skill? You don't have to be a natural or end up with Instagram-worthy dishes. Focus on the fundamentals, follow the recipes, and enjoy learning to feel more at home in your own kitchen.

For my family, the kitchen is not only where we learn to cook and eat healthfully, but also where some of our most important family conversations take place. I try to keep the environment friendly and spiritually healthy so our entire family feels welcome and free to be open and honest. For me, maintaining this open atmosphere is way more important than keeping a perfect or even clean kitchen. My motto in the kitchen is "God bless this mess!" Lord knows, if we're putting recipes together several times a day as quickly as possible, it won't be without messes. Whether it's feeding family, cooking for friends, or taking the time to cook a meal for yourself, my

# LETTING GO OF NO-CARB/LOW-CARB DIETS

Carbs can be our best friend *if* we respect them. I can't tell you how often I hear someone say they've given up carbs when what they mean is they've given up bread and pasta. So let's get something straight: Just like fat, there are beneficial carbs and not-as-beneficial carbs. When we say "carbs," we tend to think of the nonbeneficial carbs, such as processed white bread, processed snacks, and baked treats. You may not realize that many other foods fall into the carb category as well: everything from fruits, veggies, and legumes to honey and maple syrup. These are all carbs, too, and they have mega benefits in our bodies.

Carbs are essential for providing the energy your body needs. As long as you are choosing them well and pairing them with healthy fats and protein, they will allow you to get that energy throughout the day and burn fat. Still, I know it may be hard to let go of the low-carb or no-carb diets. Let me see if I can convince you naysayers out there who aren't ready to add carbs back into your lives.

## My Top 5 Reasons *Not* to Go on a Low-Carb Diet

**1.** **It's unsustainable.** Physically, your body will get tired and you will start burning muscle instead of fat for energy. There are social barriers, too. It's not easy to be on such a restricted diet that you can't go to restaurants or eat at a party.

**2.** **It can cause long-term damage.** Low energy, reduced mental capacity, anxiety, and hypoglycemia (low blood sugar) are just some of the effects of low-carb diets—not to mention that once you start eating carbs again, you may experience insulin resistance, which can lead to type 2 diabetes.

**3.** **It gives you bad breath.** Yuck! If your health is not enough to convince you, think about your poor family, friends, and co-workers. When you're not using carbs for energy, your body burns fat that releases ketones, and the chemicals in these ketones . . . stink! There is no fix for low-carb bad breath, other than balancing your diet with carbs.

**4.** **It can create organ confusion.** You need carbs, not only for the energy to exercise but also for your body to do all its daily work of functioning properly. Carbs fuel your hormone levels, temperature regulation, and digestion, just to name a few. Without them as fuel, your liver works overtime to produce ketones as a substitute fuel, and your kidneys get stressed metabolizing the amounts of protein required to offset the lack of carbs. If your liver and kidneys are stressed and overworked, they won't be able to function as intended.

**5.** **The initial weight loss boost is only water weight.** When you restrict your carb intake, you will lose some water weight, because carbs do carry water. But the effects of this weight loss are temporary. Once you've lost that initial water weight, the effect stalls out, and your weight loss plateaus.

I truly believe that weight loss really isn't all that rewarding if you don't feel good. Carbs are essential to your body and well-being. Welcome them back. You won't be sorry!

advice is to embrace the mess. The mess just shows the effort we're making to take care of our loved ones and ourselves—and isn't that a gift!

In other words, if you're used to having a clean kitchen with everything in its place but you don't cook in it very often, or work obsessively to avoid making a mess, you may want to give yourself permission to focus on the heart of your kitchen—providing food and a sense of well-being for your own health and your family's. Feel good in your kitchen!

## APPRECIATING THE PRIVILEGE OF THE OPPORTUNITY TO CREATE HEALTHY HABITS

So often, I hear people saying that the only thing they would do differently with the Feel-Good approach is that they wish they'd started sooner. But I want to remind you that timing is a part of life, and whenever you were brought to the Feel-Good Way, that is the right time for you. Be patient and loving with yourself, as the best is yet to come! Let go of any shame or guilt that created negative habits around food and embrace the goodness of real-food eating once and for all—not to look a certain way, but to feel a certain way. After just one week, you may start getting compliments about the pep in your step or the glow to your skin. After a month or so, you may need to do some shopping for a couple of new outfits! It's a process, and part of the process is trusting the system and trusting the timing of your health journey.

There's no better feeling than knowing you have the tools to prevent disease and health issues for yourself and your family. What a privilege it is to introduce this to the children in our lives as well so they can learn how good and healthful food can be without the long road the rest of us took to get here! I'm thankful for the opportunity, and so thankful to be able to share it with you.

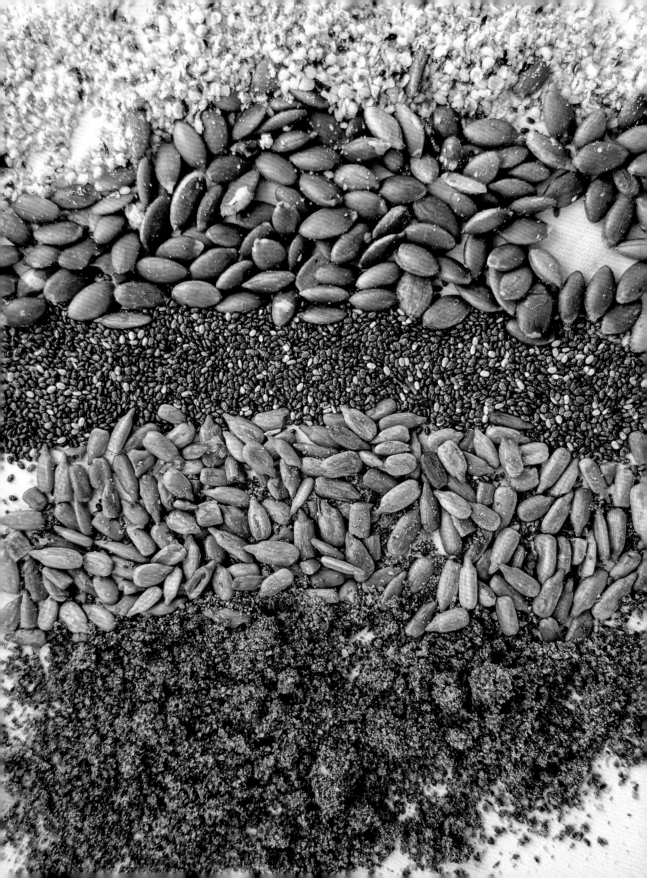

# FEEL-GOOD FRAMEWORK
## getting started

**Below I've included** tools and pantry ingredients to get your Feel-Good kitchen going. Don't feel like you need to go out and purchase all these tools and ingredients. (As you know, the Feel-Good Way is not an all-or-nothing concept.) Consider the lists below a reference of tools and ingredients that you may come across in the recipes and that you may decide you want to add to your kitchen.

## FEEL-GOOD TOOLS FOR YOUR KITCHEN

Food processor

High-powered blender

Mason jars, 1-pint and 1-quart sizes

Nontoxic pots and pans

Baking pan and muffin tin (I like silicone)

Silicone baking mat or parchment paper

Vegetable spiralizer

Milk frother (while not necessary, it's very helpful for homemade beverages)

## FEEL-GOOD FUEL

There are a handful of Feel-Good ingredients I use a lot in my recipes. Some of them you're probably familiar with and others you may not have come across before.

### ALMOND FLOUR AND ALMOND MEAL:
Almond flour and almond meal are made from ground almonds, making them gluten-free and more nutrient-dense than traditional flour. The flour and the meal are interchangeable, but each creates a slightly different consistency. For the recipes in this book, I indicate in the ingredients list whether almond flour or almond meal works best, or if you can use either. Almond flour works great for baking, but not so great for thickening soups or sauces.

> ### Feel-Good Fundamentals Reminder
>
> **1.** Combine macros—carbs, protein, and fat—when you eat.
>
> **2.** Eat within an hour of waking up, then every four hours.
>
> **3.** Eat the rainbow. Try to eat five different colors every day.
>
> **4.** Drink eighty ounces of water.
>
> **5.** Move your body four times a week for thirty minutes.

**ARROWROOT:** Arrowroot comes from a tropical plant that is part of the ginger root family. Unlike ginger, however, arrowroot has no distinct taste, which is why it works great as a thickener in place of wheat flour or cornstarch without altering the taste of the other ingredients.

**BEE POLLEN:** Bee pollen is antiviral and packed with antioxidants. Added to recipes, it increases phytonutrients the same way a superfood does. Because it's more of a beneficial additive than core ingredient, it's okay to omit bee pollen from recipes if you'd like, since it doesn't affect the macro balance.

**BONE BROTH:** You can find bone broth in the soup section of the grocery store. Unlike regular broth, which is derived from the meat of an animal, bone broth comes from the bones and has more gelatin, or collagen. This means it contains more complex protein than regular broth and helps with digestion as well. Cooking with bone broth also makes eating meat more sustainable, as nothing goes to waste. Can you substitute bone broth for any recipe that calls for chicken or beef broth? You could, but do be aware that it delivers a different nutritional profile. Bone broth has 9 grams of protein per serving while traditional chicken or beef broth has about 2 grams, making bone broth a great way to add more protein to a soup-based meal. If you don't need more protein to balance your macros, then you can choose traditional over the bone variety.

**CACAO NIBS:** These add a great crunch, texture, and slight sweetness to your desserts, smoothies, and bowls. The taste is bittersweet, kind of like crunching into the combination of dark chocolate and coffee, while packing a ton of fiber and flavonoids. Cacao nibs can be challenging to find, so you may want to purchase online to avoid frustration.

**CACAO POWDER:** Unlike *cocoa* powder, which is derived from a heating process, cacao is cold-pressed, leaving behind the most powerful nutrients. As cacao powder has become more popular, it has become easier to find. I love to buy it in bulk online, though, giving me more bang for the buck!

**CAMU-CAMU:** Similar to bee pollen, camu-camu is a bonus antioxidant that doesn't change the macros but enhances the bioavailability of nutrients we consume with our smoothies, shakes, and bowls. Camu-camu is a berry native to the rainforest. Like other berries, it is high in antioxidants, especially vitamin C, which improves immune function.

**CASSAVA FLOUR:** Cassava and tiger nut are two of my favorite lesser-known flour options for baking. Both are made from root vegetables (tiger nut is not a nut!) and both are gluten-free. None of these recipes specifically call for tiger nut flour, but tiger nut and cassava flour are interchangeable.

**CAULIFLOWER RICE:** When a recipe calls for cauliflower rice, it's not because I'm trying to replace your complex carb of real rice. I am hoping to bulk up your meals with more cruciferous veggies. Cauliflower has a light flavor when diced into rice, and it can be added to smoothies, soups, sauces, and more without altering the more dominant flavors. It's also easy to find in most stores in the freezer section, where it's already in rice form and ready to use.

**CHIA SEEDS:** More omega-3, please! Chia seeds are loaded with essential fatty acids and even carry a few grams of protein. They're great for buffing up your smoothies and balancing out the beautiful colors. Our brains and cholesterol levels will thank us for using these! White chia is harder to find, and I'd suggest purchasing it online, but black chia seeds are usually found in the baking section near the "healthy" or organic flour options.

**COCONUT AMINOS:** This condiment is similar to soy sauce, but it's much easier to digest for most people. I'm out with the soy, in with the coconut. You won't miss the flavor of soy because the taste of this alternative is very much like soy sauce and

> **Bioavailability** is a term that describes how effectively and efficiently a vitamin or nutrient is delivered to where it is most beneficial within our bodies. The more bioavailable a nutrient is, the more immediate and significant its effect on the body.

it even looks like soy sauce. Typically found in the Asian cooking section, coconut aminos flavor your stir-fries and other dishes while providing more nutrients than their lookalike cousin.

**COCONUT FLOUR:** Coconut flour helps promote a stable blood sugar. It's easy to find in the baking section, but it does take a little adjustment to bake with. It absorbs twice as much liquid as traditional flour and even gluten-free flour, so you'll need only about half of it and sometimes less when substituting with it. For the recipes in this book, follow the amount called for, and you'll be fine.

**COCONUT OIL:** Coconut oil has become a controversial ingredient over the years because of its high saturated fat, but what is unique about it is that it's made up of medium-chain triglycerides (MCTs) that offer a plethora of health benefits. I am a big fan of alternating your healthy oils. Typically, I use coconut oil or butter when baking, avocado oil or ghee when cooking, and olive oil as a dressing or for cold-to-room-temperature dishes. Coconut oil solidifies at room or cool temps, so it often needs to be melted if you're mixing it into a recipe.

**COCONUT SUGAR:** As you begin the Feel-Good approach to eating, you'll notice a change in how sugar makes you feel. Coconut sugar has more fiber and less sweetness than granulated sugar and will likely become your new best friend in baking. It's

| healthy oils | unhealthy oils |
|---|---|
| • avocado oil | • sunflower oil |
| • coconut oil | • canola oil |
| • olive oil | • vegetable oil |
| • nut and seed oils | • corn oil |
| • ghee | • grapeseed oil |
| • 100% pure oil cooking sprays | • soybean oil |
| | • safflower oil |
| | • shortening |
| | • margarine |
| | • cooking sprays (such as PAM) |

*add these*

*remove these*

easy to find in the baking section of most grocery stores.

**COLLAGEN PEPTIDES:** I'm sure you've heard about collagen, as it's been all the rage the last ten years or so—and for good reason! Collagen contains all the essential amino acids and is a protein powerhouse. It's my preferred form of protein powder for real-food smoothies, but like food, not all collagen is created equal. It's important to research where it's made and how it's sourced and to make sure there are no unnecessary additives. This is one of those products where quality can be sacrificed once it hits the huge market. So, shop small! I look for a brand that's sustainably sourced, and it's even more ideal if it comes from multiple parts of the bovine. I personally love these brands: Thorne, Revive, and Great Lakes. To make recipes that call

for collagen peptides vegetarian, you can substitute a vegetarian protein powder for the peptides.

**COOKING SPRAY:** Look for a cooking spray without unnecessary additives, such as the spray from Thrive Market. I typically use coconut or avocado oil spray because of their high smoke points.

**EXTRA-VIRGIN OLIVE OIL:** *Extra-virgin* means that the oil is the least processed form and has retained many of its antioxidants, which can be lost during processing. Our goal is to feel good and to retain as many nutrients as possible. The less processing, the more nutrition!

**FILTERED WATER:** Our water source is very important to our overall health and how we feel. Use filtered water when you can, which means pure water, without harsh chemicals like fluoride and chlorine. Whether you're cooking with it, consuming it, or even just showering with it, it's always a good idea to have your water tested to know what you're working with. If you're using city water or not sure what your water source is, you might consider a filtration system. You can also look up your location and potential contaminants using the Tap Water Database at ewg.org.

**FLAX/CHIA EGGS:** Do you have an egg intolerance or allergy? No problem! The best alternative is to make flax eggs or chia eggs instead. All you need is the seed meal and water. I use my coffee grinder to grind up the seeds so that they are as small and fluffy as possible. Combine 1 tablespoon of ground seed or meal and 3 tablespoons of water and let it sit for at least 15 minutes. Then add it to any recipe in place of 1 egg.

**FLAXSEED MEAL:** Flaxseeds are very hard for us to digest, so it's best for our bodies when they've been broken down into meal before using them in recipes. Flaxseed meal is usually found in the flour/baking section in stores. A little bit goes a long way.

**GHEE:** If you haven't tried ghee yet, you're missing out! A staple in Indian cooking, it has such a delicious and bold flavor, like the richest butter you've ever tasted. It's made by removing the milk solids from butter, which takes out the lactose and casein, leaving behind high omega-3s. It also has a high smoke point, so it's super versatile for use in the kitchen.

**GINGER:** I like to keep ginger on hand, both in fresh and powder form. Not only is ginger tasty, it aids digestion, reduces nausea, and contains antioxidant and anti-inflammatory compounds.

**HEMP HEARTS/SEEDS:** These two are not to be confused because they're the same thing! Hemp hearts/seeds, like chia and flax, are loaded with fiber and amazing fatty acids. Hemp is a little higher in protein than other seeds, helping to balance the natural sugar in our real-food smoothies.

**MACA POWDER:** Maca powder is made from a Peruvian plant that has been cultivated for more than two thousand years in the central Andes. It is high in many trace minerals and can help with metabolic and endocrine health. I've heard women say it even improved their libido. (Happy hormones!) This one can be hard to find in stores, but thankfully it's shelf-stable. I suggest buying online and then start adding it to your smoothies.

**MĀNUKA HONEY:** Mānuka honey is interchangeable with raw, organic, local honey, but it's the ultimate powerhouse. Harvested only in New Zealand, it packs a powerful antiviral, antibacterial, and anti-inflammatory punch. In fact, you could even use mānuka honey as a face mask for inflammation! It's not cheap, so I like to

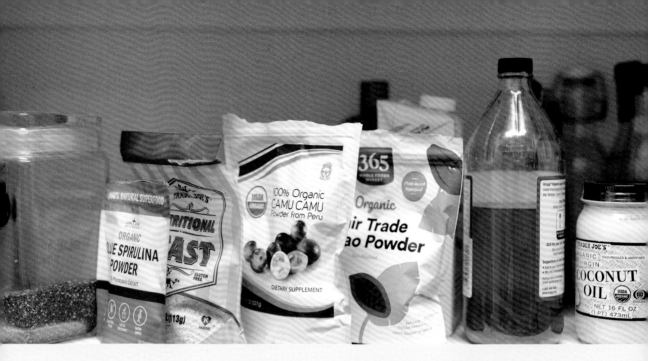

have it around for special occasions and recipes that call for less than a tablespoon.

**MAPLE SYRUP:** My clients often voice their concern over maple syrup in our recipes due to its high sugar content. Yes, the sugar content is high, but the calories from maple syrup are not empty. Maple syrup, being minimally processed, offers several essential vitamins and minerals that are bioavailable upon ingesting. Its taste is like nothing else out there, and it's my favorite swap for sugar in baking. Fear not the maple syrup, and savor its sweetness.

**MILK:** As long as your body can tolerate it, I'm good with any variety of milk. My favorites are raw dairy milk, almond milk, cashew milk, and coconut milk. Flax milk is a great alternative if you can't do nuts or dairy. Generally, I keep one dairy milk and one nut milk in the fridge.

**NUT BUTTERS:** I'm a fanatic when it comes to nut butters. They offer healthy fat and protein, so they can easily be served on the side of most carbs, making them convenient macro balancers. They are also some of my favorite foods in the world. If you have more than one on hand, nothing tastes better than a combination of nut butters in an energy bite (see pages 230 and 231). The recipes call for one butter, but you can combine multiple butters as you like. My personal favorites: creamy natural peanut butter, almond butter, and cashew butter, as well as seed butters like sunflower and tahini. Seed butters are a great substitute if you have nut allergies in your family.

**NUTRITIONAL YEAST:** Loaded with B vitamins and amino acids, nutritional yeast is a great nondairy, nonmeat alternative for adding flavor and protein to recipes.

It gives a nutty, cheesy flavor to your foods and is a great addition to keep on hand, particularly in a vegetarian kitchen.

**SALT:** Table salt is out, and I feel 100 percent comfortable letting you know that. Traditional table salt contains harmful additives—everything from anticaking agents to aluminum—and is problematic to your health. So toss all your table salt and replace it with sea salt, Himalayan pink salt, and Celtic salt. Salts such as these boast more trace minerals than anything else in nature, and these trace minerals benefit hundreds of biochemical processes in our bodies, including healthy healing and our immune system. They also aid muscle growth and neurological functioning.

**SPIRULINA/CHLORELLA POWDER:** This is another great addition to your smoothies. It doesn't taste the best, but when combined with fruit, you'll never know it's there. Spirulina helps improve the rate at which cells turn over, which means faster healing. Chlorella helps to improve collagen production. Grab it at your favorite online store.

**SPROUTED-GRAIN BREAD:** Very similar to regular bread but with sprouted grain—because while we don't stop eating bread here, we do love to digest it as well as possible. When the grains are sprouted, it removes a shell-type layer that can cause digestive issues. Without this hard shell,

we're able to utilize the nutrients from the bread faster and better. These breads are often found in the freezer section because they don't have preservatives added to keep them fresh.

**TAHINI:** Tahini is ground sesame seed butter. Not only is it a great alternative to nuts for those who are allergic, but it's actually very versatile in cooking and baking, and it improves the nutrient profile while adding protein and omega-3s. It's one of the main ingredients in hummus, but I also use tahini in brownies, sauces for lettuce wraps, and energy bites. You might be surprised to see this becoming one of your everyday staples.

**TAPIOCA STARCH:** Similar to arrowroot, tapioca starch is another great alternative to thicken up a sauce, soup, or gravy. It's interchangeable with arrowroot and cornstarch, so don't feel like you need to keep all three of them on hand.

**TURMERIC:** I love having turmeric, in fresh and powder form, on hand at all times. This is a potent anti-inflammatory ingredient, so have it ready for injury, pain, or sickness. It's also rich in phytonutrients that can neutralize free radicals in their path. Be warned, though: It's also my favorite natural food dye, so if you spill it, wipe it up quickly and wash your hands because it has a way of turning everything yellow!

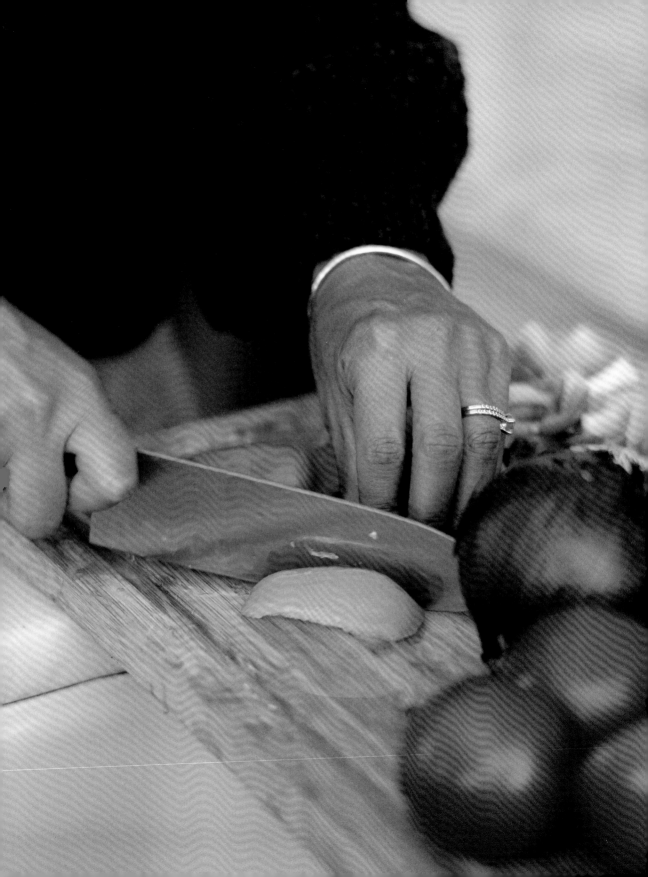

# A DAY OF
# THE FEEL-GOOD WAY

· · · · · · · · · · · · · · · · · · · · · · · · · · · · · · · · · · · · · · · · · · · · · · · · ·

## sample meal plan

*The Feel-Good fundamentals* suggest that you eat every four hours to keep your blood sugar balanced and optimal energy flowing. But how does that look in practice? I've laid out a sample meal plan, designed to keep your blood sugar stable and your body operating in a state of homeostasis. As you adopt the lifestyle of combining your macros every four hours, you'll notice how intuitive this becomes and how you won't need a reference guide. You're welcome to repeat meals while you're starting out, if that's more practical for your lifestyle, or you're welcome to mix and match with a variety of foods. The key is that you make this work for you and your lifestyle and enjoy the foods that are going to be fueling you.

> **Homeostasis** is when all our body systems are operating optimally and efficiently. Our blood sugar and our blood pressure are stable and our body is maintaining a balanced environment to do all its work, making us feel good.

**DAY ONE**

BREAKFAST
Buddha Brekkie Bowl (page 62)

LUNCH
Fermented Cucumber Salad (page 145)

SNACK
Carrots plus Garlic Hummus (page 151)
and Homemade Crackers (page 154)

DINNER
Superfood Chili (page 183)

DESSERT
Nice Cream (page 241)

**DAY TWO**

BREAKFAST
Huevos Rancheros Casserole (page 67)

SNACK
Chewy Chocolate Energy Bites
(page 230) or Cookie Dough Energy
Bites (page 231)

LUNCH
Loaded "Nachos" (page 117)

DINNER
Egg Roll Skillet (page 199)

**DAY THREE**

BREAKFAST
Super Strawberry Rhubarb Smoothie
(page 91)

LUNCH
Walnut Beet Salad (page 142)

SNACK
Stuffed Sweet Potato (page 160)

DINNER
Spring Skillet Lasagna (page 196)

**DAY FOUR**

BREAKFAST
Citrus Gingerberry Smoothie (page 97)

SNACK
Easy English Muffin (page 53)

LUNCH
Cruciferous Crunch Salad (page 146)

SNACK
Seven-Layer Dip (page 157)

DINNER
Chili Lime Chicken (page 210)

**DAY FIVE**

BREAKFAST
Key Lime Pie Smoothie (page 92)

LUNCH
Mexican Caesar Power Bowl (page 133)

SNACK
Pesto Dip with Crackers (page 154) and
veggies

DINNER
Fish Taco Slaw Bowls (page 218)

This particular schedule—smoothie breakfast, lunch, afternoon snack, and dinner—is probably the most popular setup among my clients when planning their meals for the day. Most people align with the four meals a day for scheduling as well as convenience. They also feel better than ever with a morning smoothie. For me, I love a morning smoothie, but it takes me around thirty to forty-five minutes to finish it. It's not a meal you can or should eat too quickly! So keep that in mind for your scheduling, too.

## FOR MY VEGETARIAN FRIENDS

Some vegetarians eat eggs, and some choose not to. For this book, anything I label vegetarian does not include eggs. And please note that most of the recipes can be modified to be vegetarian. When that's the case, I've made a note above the recipe. Several of the breakfast recipes contain eggs. Some won't work if you omit the eggs, but a lot of them will. Several of the smoothie recipes include collagen peptides, but these can be replaced by vegetarian protein powder. So, look for the vegetarian tag, but know that you can modify many of the other recipes in a way that works for you and your family. If additional protein is needed, I will offer you a swap. If additional protein isn't needed to fit your macros, then I will suggest simply omitting the animal protein source.

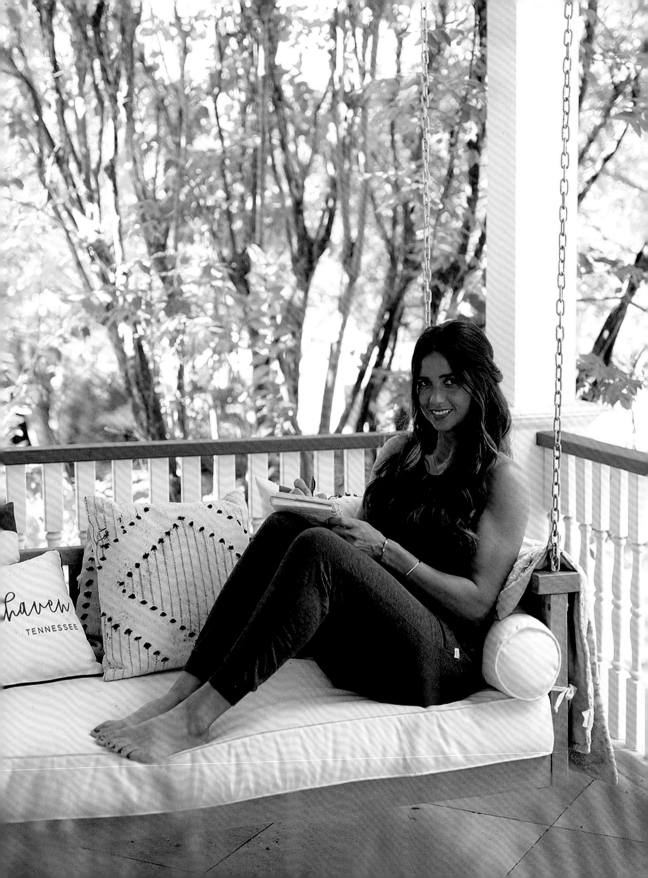

# LISTENING PRAYER
# TO BEGIN THE DAY

***A big part*** of my Feel-Good Way (and life!) is prayer. A few years ago, I started sharing prayer with my CCN community and asking for prayer requests on social media. Then I started implementing it in my challenge programs. The first time I did, the feedback was incredible. During live sessions on Zoom, I could see the tears flowing as people relaxed their systems more than they were used to.

Healing with prayer isn't the same instant gratification as, say, eating a macro-balanced meal that provides energy. But it does impact your central nervous system, sometimes instantly. When you pray, you surrender the control and worry you feel over your life, an act that almost always reduces the stress you're carrying. Prayer institutes a faith higher than yourself, whose benefits only grow stronger every day.

I never want to force someone to adopt my beliefs, but I do want to present these practices as a way to improve our health and our lives. So in this book, I've included prayers throughout the chapters to encourage you and support you in checking in with your spiritual and emotional health. I hope these prayers and practices can nourish your soul as you're nourishing your body every day.

My favorite form of prayer is called listening prayer. Each morning, I make a point of sitting in silence and peace and trying to seek God's purpose. I try to do this for at least fifteen minutes, but it really depends on the day. Here's how I usually proceed through my listening prayer:

I sit in a chair with my back straight, but relaxed. I put my palms on my knees, facing up toward heaven, ready to receive blessing. I imagine my feet planted firmly in the ground and my head gently being pulled toward heaven. I think about relaxing my face and body. I close my eyes and unclench my jaw and mouth.

I imagine myself at the lake—one of

the places I feel most at ease—with all its sights, sounds, smells, and sensations and its peaceful expanse of water.

In a minimal number of words, I begin my listening prayer by saying, *Lord, I consecrate this day to you.*

I consecrate each of my family members and call them out by name, including myself. I consecrate any projects with work and the people associated with them. I ask the Lord to use me as a vessel to grow his kingdom and reflect his love through me.

Then I sit and listen for at least ten minutes. I never leave my imaginary spot while I'm listening to what he wants to tell me.

At the end of the time period, I write down anything I want to remember. I don't experience an epiphany about my family, friends, or work every single day. But I do consistently leave those prayers feeling complete peace and surrender, even if my schedule is beyond overwhelming. I thrive when I start my morning this way, and sometimes, especially in heightened or stressful times, I come back to it at lunch or in the afternoon.

I need this practice as much as I need the water I drink and the air I breathe. If I don't make time for it, I feel a constant sense of overwhelm. Listening prayer is relaxing, and, beyond that, it helps me schedule my day in a way that points back to my kingdom assignment—God's plan for me. Sometimes I hear whispers and his voice in guidance, and other times I just feel a sense of what is serving him and what is not.

No matter what worldview you come from, this practice can be of great value. It benefits the nervous system, which then impacts your mental and emotional health, which impacts your sleep, which impacts your overall well-being. I have noticed spiritual neglect in so many people who come to me seeking health or healing, so I include my personal faith and practices as elements you may want to adapt in your own way to impact your life. Faith in something outside of your own control, whatever form that takes for you, is a powerful force that can be transformative to our daily existence, our purpose, and our lives.

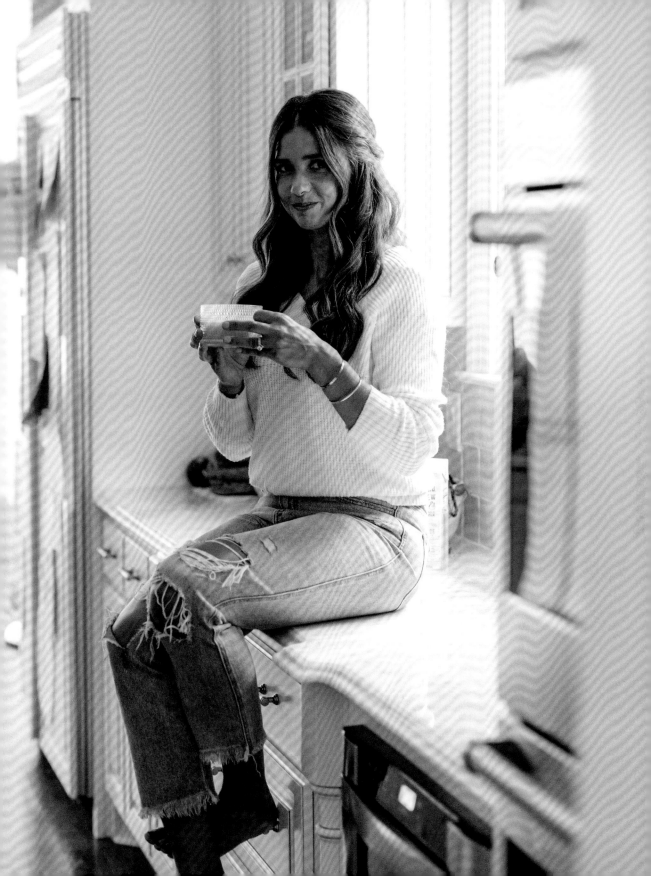

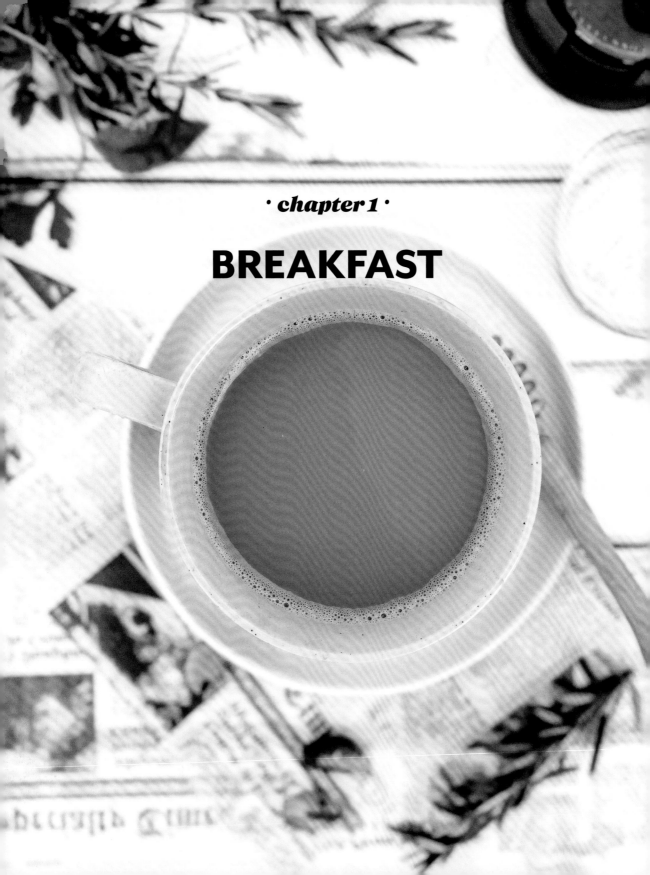

· *chapter 1* ·

# BREAKFAST

. . . . . . . . . . . . . . . . . . . . .

**When we eat** breakfast each morning, we are literally breaking the fast. That first bite of food signals to our bodies that it's time to start burning energy. Our growth hormones become active, then the liver wakes up, then the endocrine system. We're activating our energy cycle. Soon, cells are turning over in our system, and our body is ready to burn calories from our stored fuel and food.

When we *don't* eat breakfast, our bodies go into reverse-psychology mode. The body thinks we don't need any energy, so it stores energy in our reserves instead of burning it, interfering with our cortisol levels (that's the stress hormone) along the way. Nobody wants extra stored energy or crazy cortisol levels to start the day! When we eat a healthy breakfast, however, we are letting our body know we're going to nourish it with energy for the whole day. It's like giving ourselves a reassuring morning hug.

I know mornings can be *very* hectic! But when we make time to eat a healthy breakfast—and, when we can, eat it together as a family—we are starting the day in unity and nourishment, ready to face whatever comes our way.

I like to say a little prayer as I'm sitting down with my morning coffee or tea, before everyone else is up and at the breakfast table. It keeps me from feeling like I'm taking on the weight of the world. It usually goes something like this . . .

*Oh God,* I consecrate this day to you. I surrender every minute and every opportunity to you. I take a moment this morning to reflect on the goodness of this day. As the sun has risen again, I'm given another day to grow for myself and my family. I'm so grateful for another day. Bless the meals I prepare to provide my body nourishment all the way into my cells. Bless my appetite to be satisfied and in union with my health goals. Bless my home and my family with optimal health. I'm so thankful for the gift of health and a home and family to share that with. In the depth of my heart, I feel so close to my health goals. Thank you for that. We pray in your name. Amen.

Every day is a new chance. Every meal is a new opportunity. How will you make today count? Let's start with breakfast!

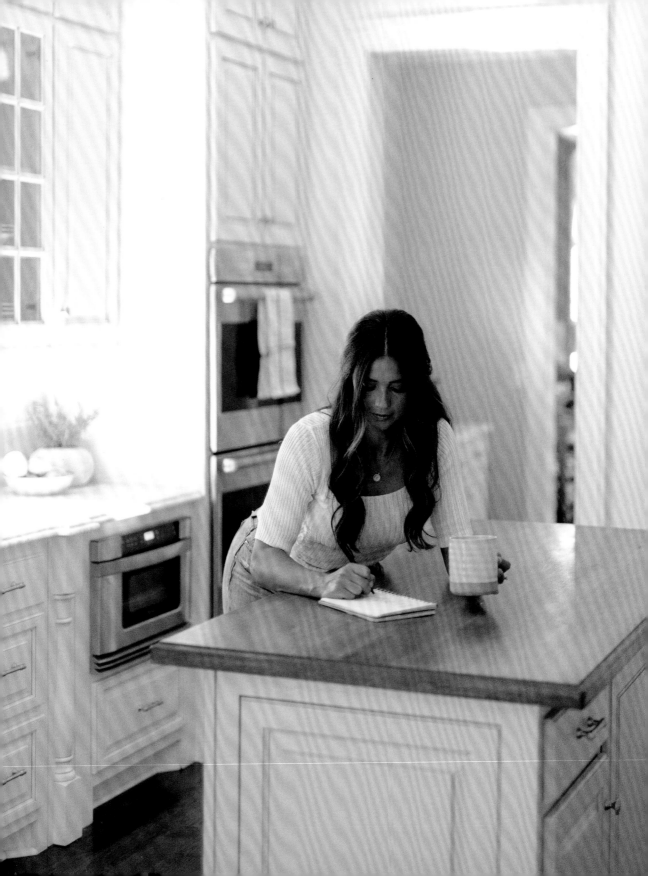

# EASY ENGLISH MUFFIN

*I*f you're anything like me, "quick and convenient" is a huge priority in the morning. This recipe fits the bill, and it's delicious, inviting you to add colorful toppings, such as berries or whatever fruit is in season. You could also spice it up with a little pumpkin and pumpkin pie spice. You only need a couple of minutes to make this breakfast a delicious part of your morning.

SERVES 1

. . . . . . . . . . . . . . . . . . . . . .

1 banana

1 egg

1 tablespoon unsweetened nut milk (such as almond or cashew), coconut milk, or flax milk

⅓ cup almond flour

¼ teaspoon baking powder

1 tablespoon natural nut or seed butter (such as cashew, almond, peanut, or sunflower seed), for serving

¼ cup berries, for serving

Preheat the oven to 350°F.

In a small bowl, mash the banana and mix in the egg and milk. Stir well until smooth. Add the flour and baking powder, mix well, and pour the mixture into a small ovenproof bowl or ramekin. Bake until a toothpick comes out clean, about 20 minutes. (Alternatively, place in a microwave-safe bowl and microwave for 3 minutes.)

Let the muffin cool slightly, then dump it out of the bowl. Slice it down the middle and toast. Add the nut butter and berries to serve.

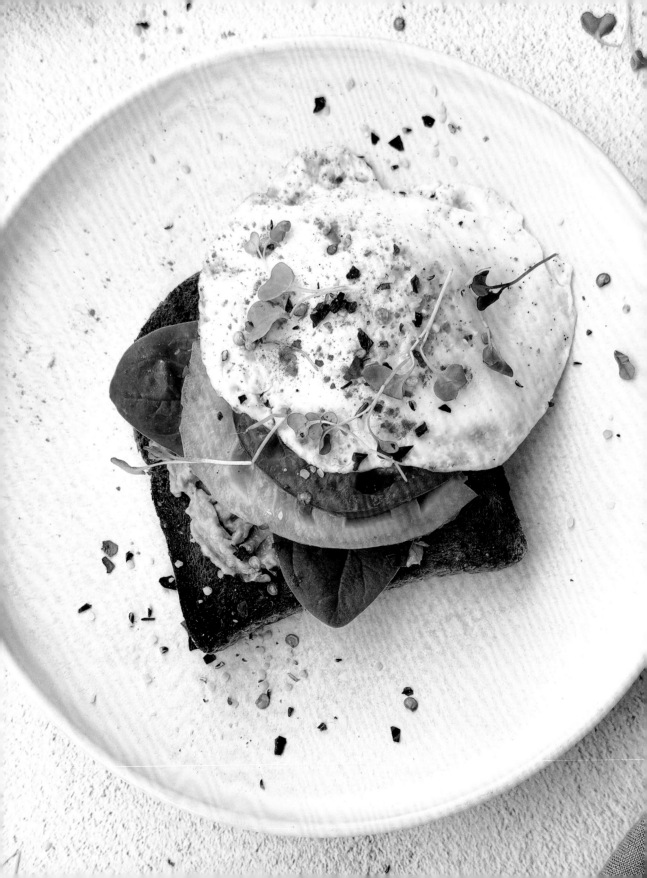

# AVOCADO TOAST

*Y*ou don't have to spend fourteen dollars at a restaurant to enjoy avocado toast. This is one of my all-time favorite breakfasts, to the point where it's hard for me to feel satisfied at breakfast without the filling nature of the healthy fat in avocado. If you're feeling zesty, you can also spritz a little lemon or other citrus over the top.

**SERVES 1**

TO MAKE VEGETARIAN, OMIT THE EGGS.

1 slice sprouted whole-grain bread (such as Ezekiel or Dave's Killer Bread)

¼ avocado

Sprinkle of red pepper flakes

Sprinkle of hemp seeds

Small handful of spinach

Sliced tomato

2 eggs, cooked however you like

Turmeric

Sea salt and freshly ground black pepper

Microgreens (optional), for garnish

Toast the bread. Spread and smash the avocado evenly over the toast. Sprinkle with red pepper flakes and hemp seeds. Layer the spinach, tomato slices, and eggs on top. Season the eggs with turmeric, salt, and black pepper. If desired, garnish with microgreens.

# HOMEMADE EVERYTHING BAGELS

*L*et's consider this recipe more of a weekender! It takes a little more time than most of the other breakfast recipes, but the good news is that these bagels freeze well and they're typically a family favorite. If you've never tried cassava flour before, you're in for a treat. It's high in B vitamins, so if you notice an improvement in your energy after eating this bagel, that isn't just a coincidence—it's the bioavailability of the B vitamins.

**MAKES 4 BAGELS**

1 cup cassava flour

1 cup arrowroot or tapioca starch

¼ cup avocado oil

2 tablespoons pure maple syrup

1 tablespoon filtered water

1 teaspoon baking powder

Pinch of sea salt

5 eggs

Everything bagel seasoning (such as Trader Joe's)

Preheat the oven to 350°F. Line a baking sheet with parchment paper.

Fill a soup pot with water and bring to a boil.

In a blender or food processor, combine the cassava flour, arrowroot, avocado oil, maple syrup, water, baking powder, salt, and 4 of the eggs. Blend to mix. Transfer the dough to a medium bowl and use your hands to form a ball. Separate the dough into four equal parts and form them into bagel shapes.

Once the water is boiling, gently drop the bagels into the pot, one by one. Let the bagels boil until they float to the top, about 1 minute. Transfer them to the prepared baking sheet.

In a small bowl, whisk the remaining egg and use a pastry or basting brush to brush each bagel top with the egg. Sprinkle the bagel seasoning over the bagels.

Bake until golden brown, 23 to 25 minutes.

> **How much is a pinch?** A pinch refers to that tiny amount of an ingredient that you could pick up and hold between your thumb and forefinger, about $\frac{1}{16}$ teaspoon.

# FEEL-GOOD FAQ

. . . . . . . . . . . . . . . . . . . . . . . . . . . . . . . . . . . . . . . . . . . . . . . . . . . . . . .

**So many people swear by intermittent fasting. I'm torn between trying it and committing to eating breakfast every day . . .**

Hear me out on why I'm not a fan of intermittent fasting. The Feel-Good food philosophy has a lot to do with protecting and managing your hormones so that they work for you rather than against you. When we break our fast after waking, we are telling our brains that we are up and ready to start burning fat as fuel. When we wake up and don't break our fast, particularly if we start our day with caffeine, we are telling our brains we need stress hormones to fuel our body.

Unless you are fasting for spiritual reasons, there isn't any reason to get your energy from stress hormones instead of burning fat. Why deprive or starve yourself for results that may show up on a scale but don't result in feeling good? I have had many clients come to me after trying intermittent fasting for weight loss. Some of them did lose weight—but not all of them did. Some even gained weight. What I heard most was that they didn't feel good and that their skin, hair, and sleep all suffered.

A healthy breakfast fuels our body as nature intended and supports all our hormones in a way that engages our physical and mental well-being. So, try these recipes and let yourself feel nourished and full in the morning. Why game the perfect system Mother Nature has given us by cheating ourselves out of delicious, nourishing food?

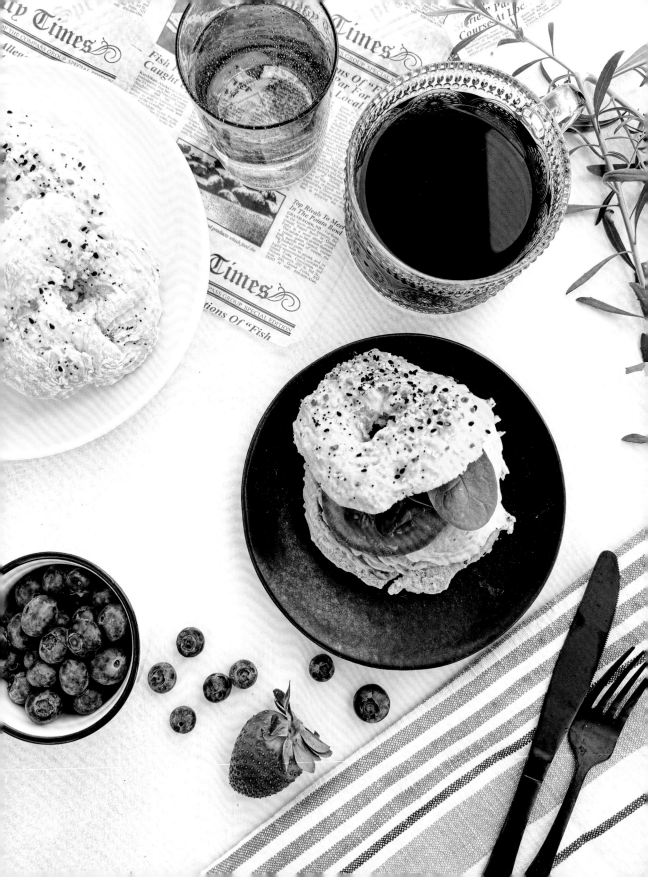

# LOADED BAGEL SANDWICH

*Y*ou don't have to give up breakfast sandwiches in order to achieve your desired health goals. Creating nutrient-dense variations of our old favorites is what really helps us develop lifestyle habits that are sustainable. Our goal is obviously to flood our bodies with nutrients, but we don't want to take the pleasure out of eating. Metabolism involves various chemical processes happening at the same time, and the feeling of pleasure can actually contribute to a healthy metabolism!

**SERVES 1**

TO MAKE VEGETARIAN, OMIT THE EGGS.

1 Homemade Everything Bagel (page 56) or store-bought gluten-free bagel (such as Outside the Breadbox)

¼ avocado

Handful of spinach

2 eggs, cooked however you like

Sliced tomato

Everything bagel seasoning (such as Trader Joe's)

½ cup berries, for serving

Toast the bagel halves. Spread and smash the avocado over one bagel half. Add the spinach, eggs, tomato, and bagel seasoning. Top with the other bagel half. Serve with the berries on the side.

# EASY BREAKFAST WRAP

**A**s much as I wish I made everything from scratch, including the gluten-free tortillas used in this wrap, I don't have the time. I have four incredibly active kids, and I want to share honestly what we do in our home. Thankfully, there are some amazing tortilla brands on the market, such as Siete. If you're in a stage of life when you have time, I encourage you to make tortillas from scratch, as they're delicious. But if you're in a hurry like me, you may come to rely on some of my store-bought favorites.

**SERVES 1**

· · · · · · · · · · · · · · · · · · · · · · ·

TO MAKE VEGETARIAN, OMIT THE EGG.

1 burrito-size grain-free tortilla (such as Siete)

1 hard-boiled egg, sliced

½ small avocado, sliced or smashed

1 cup spinach (or more), steamed

¼ cup sliced tomato

1 green onion, diced

In a skillet, warm the tortilla over medium heat for about 1 minute. Remove from the skillet and add the egg, avocado, spinach, tomato, and green onion to the tortilla. Roll up burrito-style or fold over quesadilla-style.

# ARUGULA POWER BOWL

*I* bet you're thinking, *Arugula for breakfast?* Yes! Trust me here. This is my homemade take on a veggie-boosting breakfast from the menu of one of my favorite SoCal restaurants. You might be surprised how good you feel when you start your day with this much nutrient density. Flooding your body with nutrients is a great way to support your health and longevity. Our goal is to make the process enjoyable, energizing, and satisfying.

**SERVES 1**

TO MAKE VEGETARIAN, OMIT THE EGGS.

½ cup coleslaw or broccoli slaw mix

⅓ cup cooked ancient grain (such as bulgur, farro, quinoa, or amaranth)

2 cups baby arugula

1 tablespoon crumbled goat or feta cheese (optional)

1 lemon, halved

Sea salt and freshly ground black pepper

2 eggs, cooked over easy

In a skillet, lightly heat the coleslaw over medium heat for 1 to 2 minutes. Add the cooked grains and stir to combine. Remove the skillet from the heat and let it cool slightly.

Place the arugula in a bowl. Top with the slaw mixture and cheese (if using). Squeeze the lemon over all and season with salt and pepper. Top with the eggs.

# BUDDHA BREKKIE BOWL

*I*f I had the time, I would have this meal every single morning. If you're a meal-prepper—the type of person who precuts vegetables and roasts them on Sunday night for quick and easy access during the week—this could be a super-quick meal for you. Unfortunately, my brain has never worked that way. I always have a fridge and pantry full of ingredients and options, but they're rarely prepped ahead of time unless they're leftovers from another meal. That being said, this can be a 5-minute meal if you prep ahead of time, and it's soooo worth it!

**SERVES 2**

TO MAKE VEGETARIAN, OMIT
THE EGGS.

1 tablespoon extra-virgin
    olive oil

1 medium sweet potato,
    scrubbed and diced

¼ cup diced red onion

1 garlic clove, minced

Sea salt and freshly ground
    black pepper

5 mushrooms, sliced

1 cup fresh spinach or kale

1 cup cooked quinoa

2 eggs, soft-boiled and
    halved

4 tablespoons Tahini
    Sauce (recipe follows)

½ avocado, sliced

Chopped fresh parsley, for
    serving

In a large sauté pan, heat the olive oil over medium-high heat. Add the sweet potato, onion, and garlic and cook, turning regularly, until the vegetables are softened and browned, 15 to 20 minutes. Season with salt and pepper.

Add the mushrooms and spinach and cook for another 5 minutes, or until the mushrooms are tender. Set the pan aside, keeping it warm.

Divide the quinoa and then the sweet potato mixture between two bowls and place an egg on top of each. Drizzle with the tahini sauce and top with the avocado and chopped parsley.

## TAHINI SAUCE

MAKES ¾ CUP

½ cup tahini

2 tablespoons extra-virgin olive oil

Grated zest and juice of 1 orange

2 tablespoons raw honey

2 tablespoons water

1 garlic clove, peeled but whole

Sea salt and freshly ground black pepper

In a blender, combine the tahini, olive oil, orange zest, orange juice, honey, water, and garlic and blend until smooth. Season to taste with salt and pepper. Store in an airtight container for up to 1 week in the refrigerator.

## FEEL-GOOD STORY

· · · · · · · · · · · · · · · · · · · · · · · · · · · · · · · · · · · · · · · · · · · · · · · · · · ·

### *Flannery*

When Flannery came to CCN, she was skeptical. She was a self-described "lifelong calorie-counting, carb-hating, fat-fearing dieter." She thought of food and exercise as a transaction—calories in with food, calories out with exercise, and at the end of the day, there was a correct number for success. If she missed that number or ate the "wrong" thing, she'd immediately feel bad about herself and feel further from her health goals, starting a downward emotional spiral.

After the pandemic, she discovered new forms of exercise that she really liked. She went after them with a vengeance, putting herself through grueling workouts without adjusting what she was eating to fuel her body. She actually loved how her body was looking—but how she felt was a different story. She was exhausted, she had pain in her hips and knees, and she hobbled around when she wasn't working out. At night she often woke up in pain. She didn't want to push herself so hard, but she was afraid to stop. What if she gained weight or didn't like how her body looked?

When she found CCN and the Feel-Good Way philosophy, she was excited but scared because she had tried and failed diets so many times before. She eased herself into the process of real food, eating more than she was used to and trusting the system. After only one week, she felt like a new person. She enjoyed the food she was eating. She had more energy throughout the day from eating according to a real-food philosophy that wasn't restricting her energy (calories). She slept so much better and felt more rested when she woke up. As time went on, she felt like she was losing weight, but didn't care to weigh herself anymore because she felt so good. For the first time she understood what it felt like to truly take care of her body. She felt so free, like she'd escaped a defeating cycle of tracking calories in and out. Her happiness was no longer attached to those numbers at the end of every day.

I share her story because it reminds us that the number of calories we count or the number on the scale doesn't really matter when we don't *feel* good. Learning to listen to herself, to trust herself was empowering for Flannery. I hope it can be for you, too!

Here's what she had to say: "Thank you from the bottom of my (healthier!) heart for helping me unlock the shackles that have bound me to measuring my happiness by the numbers for years. Thank you for giving me the tools to start over at thirty-nine and prepare to be my best self the rest of my life."

# VEGGIE OMELET WAFFLE

*H*ave you ever struggled with the flip of the omelet? Your omelet looks perfect for 90 percent of the cooking time, then bam, it's more like scrambled eggs? This recipe will resolve that problem and any stress associated with it! I got into making eggs on the waffle iron when we were doing a kitchen remodel and I was short on appliances. Now at our house it's a regular fun spin on a traditional omelet. Use as much bell pepper, onion, and broccoli as you'd like. You can't eat too much of these, so add to your personal preference—or feel free to switch them out for whatever veggies you're craving or have on hand.

**SERVES 1**

2 eggs

2 tablespoons water

Multicolored bell peppers, chopped

Yellow onion, chopped

Broccoli florets, chopped

Sea salt and freshly ground black pepper

Avocado or coconut oil cooking spray

Chopped tomato, for topping

¼ avocado, chopped, for topping

Yellow or green onion (optional), chopped, for topping

Sprouts (optional), for topping

Salsa or hot sauce (optional), for serving

Preheat a waffle iron.

In a small bowl, beat the eggs with the water. Add the bell peppers, onion, and broccoli and season with salt and black pepper. Coat the waffle iron with cooking spray (see Note). Add the egg and veggie mixture to the waffle iron and cook until the eggs are firm.

Serve topped with the chopped tomato and avocado. If desired, add more onion and the sprouts and serve with salsa.

**NOTE:** Before cooking the omelet, spray the waffle iron very, very well with cooking spray!

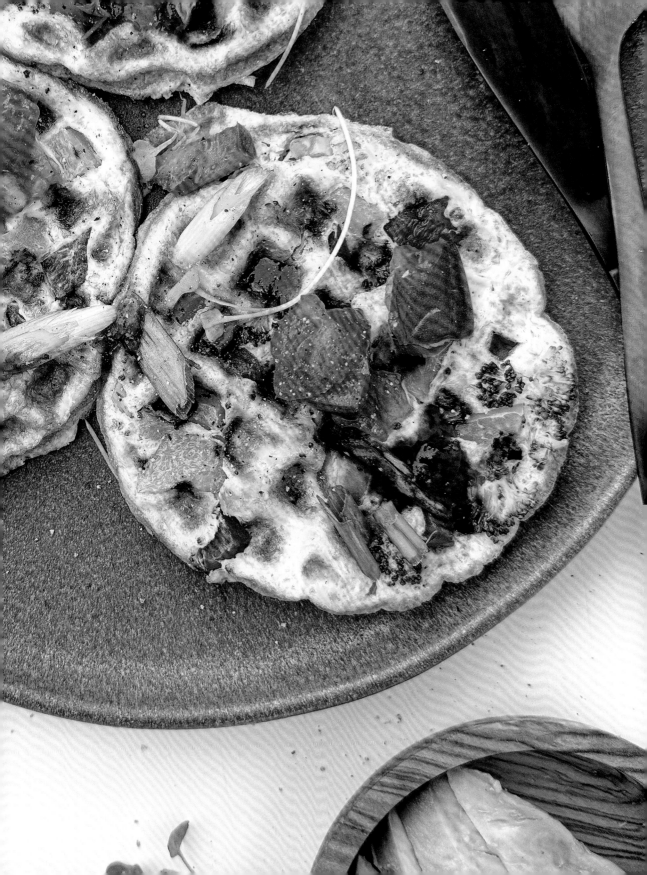

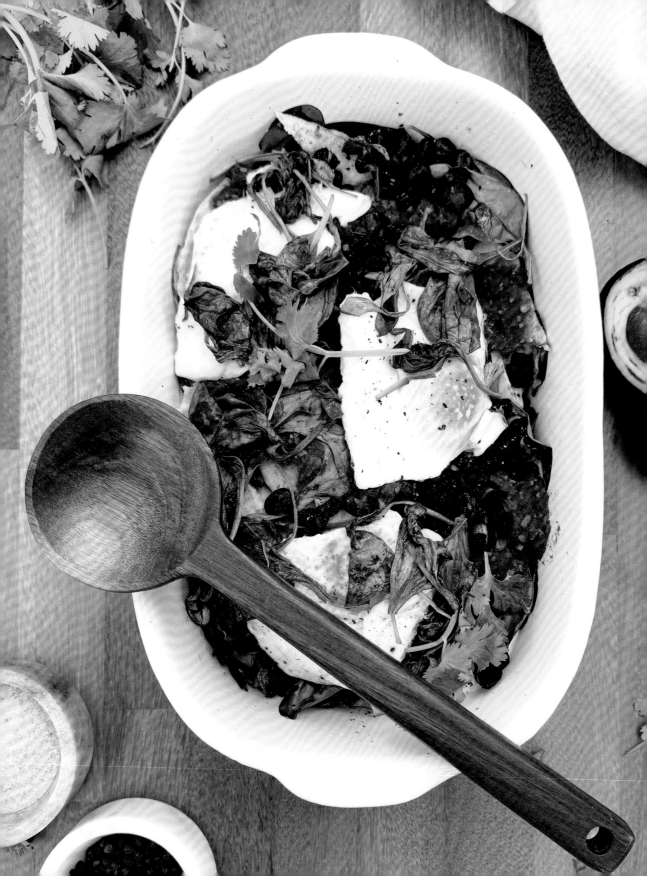

# HUEVOS RANCHEROS CASSEROLE

*I*f you're doing a shared vacation home or time with extended family, I highly recommend making this dish for breakfast. It's a fan favorite and makes plenty to serve a crowd. It's also great as leftovers! Not to mention, it's high in fiber, which means it's filling and will satiate you until your next meal. Leftovers will last in the fridge for a few days, too, so if you're not sharing with a big group, simply heat and repeat to make for easy weekday mornings.

SERVES 6 TO 8

Avocado oil cooking spray

8 grain-free flour tortillas (such as Siete)

12 eggs

1 cup canned organic black beans

1½ cups salsa

2 cups baby spinach

Sea salt and freshly ground black pepper

Avocado slices (optional), for topping

Chopped fresh cilantro (optional), for topping

Preheat the oven to 350°F. Grease a 9 by 13-inch baking dish with avocado oil spray.

Add 4 of the tortillas to the bottom of the dish. If needed, you can break them to make them fit. Crack and drop 6 eggs on top of the tortillas. Then layer ½ cup of the black beans, ¾ cup of the salsa, and 1 cup of the spinach. Season with salt and pepper to taste. Repeat the steps for a second layer, beginning with a layer of the 4 remaining tortillas.

Bake until the eggs are fully cooked to your taste, 18 to 22 minutes.

If desired, serve topped with avocado and cilantro.

# QUINOA EGG BITES

*E*gg bites are perfect for making ahead, storing in an airtight container in the refrigerator, and then popping in the microwave for a few seconds on your way out the door. They're versatile enough to eat for any meal. I love breakfast any time of day!

**SERVES 4**

Coconut oil (optional), for the muffin tin

6 eggs

1 cup cooked quinoa

½ cup chopped mushrooms

Large handful of spinach, chopped

¼ cup chopped mixed bell peppers

¼ cup chopped onion

1 cup goat cheese

Sea salt and freshly ground black pepper

Preheat the oven to 350°F. Line 12 cups of a muffin tin with silicone muffin cups or grease the muffin tin very well with coconut oil.

In a large bowl, whisk the eggs. Add the quinoa, mushrooms, spinach, bell peppers, onion, ¾ cup of the goat cheese, and salt and black pepper to taste. Stir to combine. Pour the batter into the muffin cups, dividing the batter evenly. Sprinkle the remaining ¼ cup goat cheese over the top.

Bake until the bites are golden brown and a knife inserted into the middle of one comes out clean, 18 to 22 minutes. Remove from the pan and cool.

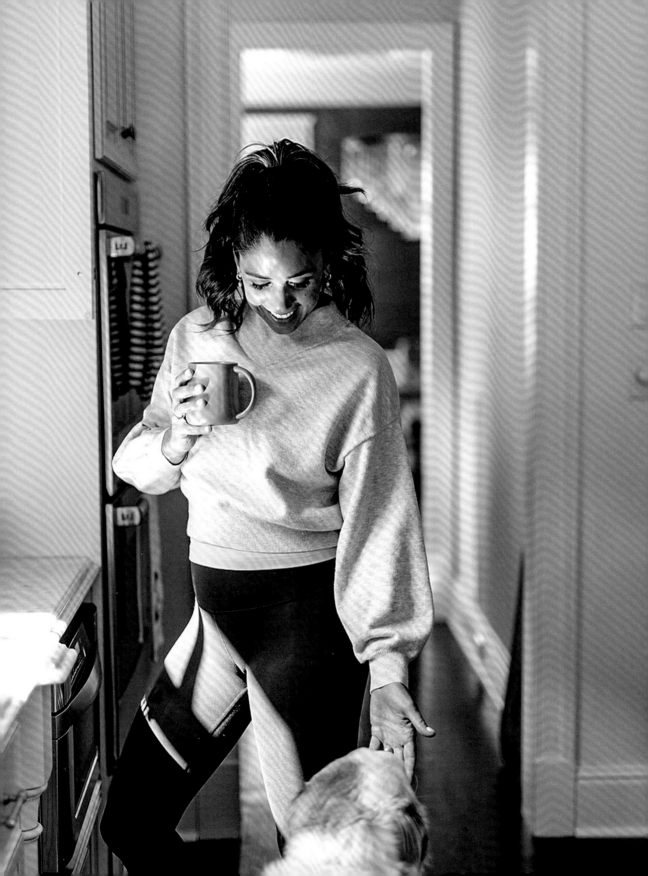

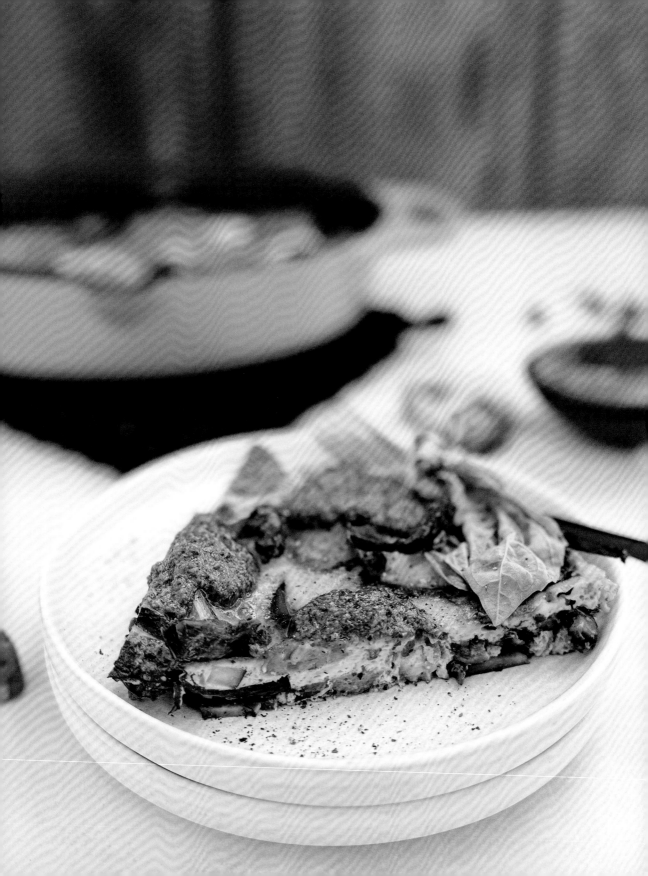

# CAST-IRON SKILLET FRITTATA

*M*y girls love this dish and ask for it regularly. For some reason, I used to make it only on holidays, but now it's part of our regular rotation. You can get creative with the ingredients by using the vegetables that are in season or leftover in your fridge. You can also omit the meat and add ¼ cup nutritional yeast and ¼ cup beans in its place.

**SERVES 4 TO 6**

3 links natural turkey or chicken breakfast sausage, sliced

1 tablespoon coconut oil or grass-fed butter

1 cup sliced Baby Bella mushrooms

1½ cups chopped kale or spinach

2 medium zucchini, spiralized into noodles, or 3 cups cooked spaghetti squash

¼ cup julienned dry-pack sun-dried tomatoes

½ teaspoon onion powder

½ teaspoon garlic powder

6 eggs, beaten

Sea salt and freshly ground black pepper

⅓ cup prepared basil pesto (I like Trader Joe's refrigerated version)

Preheat the oven to 375°F.

In a medium cast-iron skillet, cook the sausages on medium heat until lightly browned, about 8 minutes. Remove from the skillet and set aside on a plate lined with paper towels.

On medium heat, melt the coconut oil in the skillet. Add the mushrooms and cook for 2 minutes. Then add the kale, zucchini, sun-dried tomatoes, onion powder, and garlic powder. Cook until the greens are just wilted, about 5 minutes.

Pour the eggs over the veggie mixture, distributing evenly. Season with salt and pepper and let it cook for 2 minutes, allowing the eggs to set on the bottom.

Transfer to the oven and bake until a knife inserted into the center comes out clean, 20 to 25 minutes. When the frittata is done, cut it into slices and serve immediately, each topped with 1 to 2 tablespoons of pesto. Serve the cooked sausages on the side.

# SIMPLE OVERNIGHT OATS

*I* would guess this isn't your first time hearing about overnight oats. You probably already know what a versatile, fun, and delicious breakfast option this is. You probably also already know you can make every flavor you can imagine by adding whatever fresh fruit you like or frozen berries. Enjoy making these the way you love them most.

**SERVES 1**
............................

TO MAKE VEGETARIAN,
USE VEGETARIAN PROTEIN
POWDER INSTEAD OF
COLLAGEN PEPTIDES.

¾ cup rolled oats or
   gluten-free oats

¾ cup unsweetened nut
   milk

½ banana, sliced

2 tablespoons chia seeds

2 tablespoons slivered
   almonds

½ teaspoon pure vanilla
   extract

½ teaspoon pumpkin
   pie spice or ground
   cinnamon

1 scoop collagen peptides

In a 1-pint jar, combine the oats, milk, banana, chia seeds, almonds, vanilla, pumpkin pie spice, and collagen peptides. Stir if you'd like, then put the top on the jar and refrigerate overnight. Serve cool or warm the next morning in a small saucepan on the stovetop or in the microwave.

# LEMON BERRY SKILLET SCONES

$\mathcal{S}$cones . . . but easier. You don't have to shape the dough to enjoy a delicious and gluten-free scone. Since these are baked in a skillet, you cut out a lot of the legwork. I personally love lemon, whether it's in a savory or sweet recipe. These scones are just minimally sweet and so enjoyable, filling, and satisfying!

**SERVES 8**

VEGETARIAN

1½ cups raw cashews

¼ cup arrowroot flour

1 teaspoon baking powder

½ teaspoon baking soda

Pinch of sea salt

¼ cup coconut oil, melted

3 tablespoons pure maple syrup or raw honey

1½ teaspoons pure vanilla extract

1 egg or 1 flax/chia egg (see page 39)

Grated zest and juice of 1 lemon

½ cup diced fresh strawberries

½ cup frozen blueberries

Preheat the oven to 350°F. Line an 8-inch cast-iron skillet with parchment paper.

In a food processor, blend the cashews until they reach a powdery consistency, being careful not to overprocess and turn them into cashew butter. Transfer to a large bowl. Add the flour, baking powder, baking soda, and salt and whisk to combine.

In a small bowl, whisk together the coconut oil, maple syrup, vanilla, egg, lemon zest, and lemon juice. Stir the wet ingredients into the cashew mixture until well incorporated. Pour the batter into the prepared cast-iron skillet. Lightly place the strawberries and blueberries all over the top of the batter.

Bake until the edges are golden brown and a toothpick comes out clean, 26 to 30 minutes.

Let it cool for at least 15 minutes before slicing and serving.

# PEACH BERRY COBBLER OVERNIGHT OATS

*H*ere's another variation of overnight oats with endless options. You can sub in any fruit that's in season and any spice that you love. You can mix and match the nuts and seeds or you could fall in love with one version and have it on repeat! I could eat anything out of a mason jar because the jars are so cute, but of course, you could use a bowl or other container with a lid instead.

**SERVES 1**

VEGETARIAN

½ cup rolled oats or gluten-free oats

1 tablespoon chia seeds

2 tablespoons chopped pecans

½ teaspoon pure vanilla extract

¼ to ½ teaspoon ground cinnamon

¾ cup unsweetened coconut milk or nut milk

1 peach, chopped

½ cup blackberries or blueberries

In a 1-pint jar, combine the oats, chia seeds, pecans, vanilla, cinnamon, and milk. Stir until well combined. Top with the peaches and blackberries, put the top on the jar, and refrigerate overnight. Serve cool or warm the next morning in a saucepan on the stovetop or in the microwave.

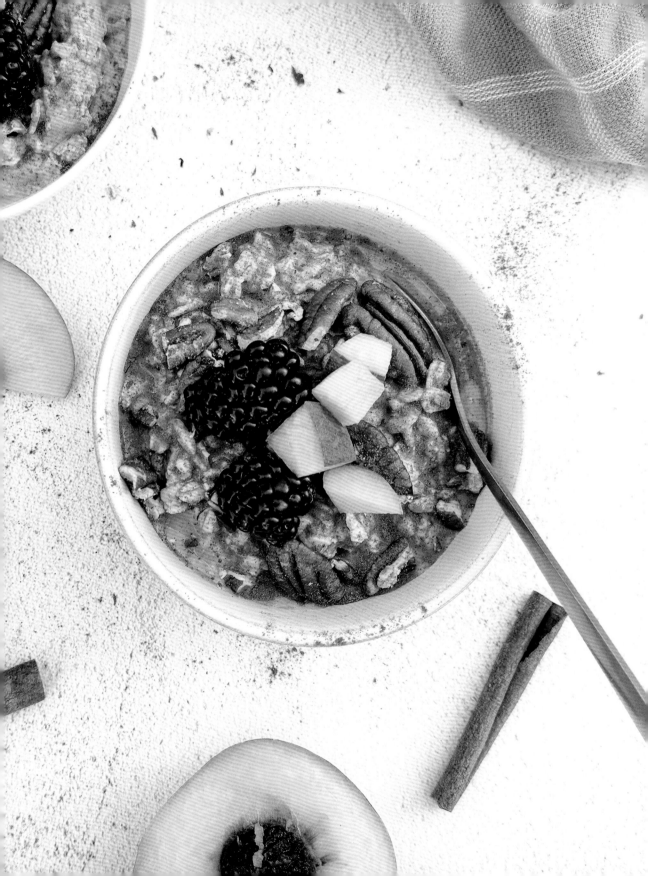

# FEEL-GOOD FAQ

........................................................................................................

### Do I have to give up my morning coffee?

Coffee has been a part of my morning routine since I was nineteen years old. I would never ask anyone to eliminate something that I haven't eliminated myself! But there are some factors to consider
since caffeine is a stimulant, meaning it speeds up the central nervous system.

- It's a good idea to eat a little something before you start guzzling. My personal hack is adding
  MCT oil and collagen peptides to my mug, so I'm getting in some healthy fat and protein while
  enjoying my morning coffee. I add half a scoop of collagen and 1 tablespoon of MCT oil. MCT
  oil is a "medium-chain triglyceride," and research shows it can improve our cognitive function,
  energy, and ability to burn fat for energy. I also eat two Brazil nuts each day with my morning
  coffee. Brazil nuts are high in selenium, a mineral that supports healthy thyroid function, but
  you don't need to eat a lot of them to make a difference. Only a couple does the trick!

- Savor and enjoy that first cup so you can maximize the experience, rather than drinking coffee
  all day or having more coffee in the afternoon. Afternoon coffee can really affect the quality of
  your sleep. Try a healthy snack instead of an afternoon coffee if you need a pick-me-up.

- Choose your coffee wisely. Coffee beans are some of the most likely crops to be sprayed with
  pesticides. Make sure the coffee you choose is organic and sustainably produced if you consume it regularly.

- The biggest problem I see with coffee is not the coffee or the amount, but what people add
  to it. A little sweetener goes a long way. My personal and professional preference to sweeten
  a cup of morning motivation is local, raw, or mānuka honey. While there are several good
  creamers on the market, it's best to keep it simple without any harmful additives. Organic
  cream or organic half-and-half are great if you crave some cream. My favorite creamy addition is Laird Superfood Adaptogen creamer. Adaptogenic mushrooms with coffee are shown
  to improve focus and hormones related to stress, such as cortisol.

- If you want to cut out caffeine but don't want to give up your warm morning drink routine,
  there are plenty of alternatives that can provide health benefits. You could try Swiss water-
  process coffee, which is truly and naturally decaffeinated coffee. Many herbal teas are decaffeinated as well. Green and black teas have many proven benefits and are lower in caffeine
  than coffee.

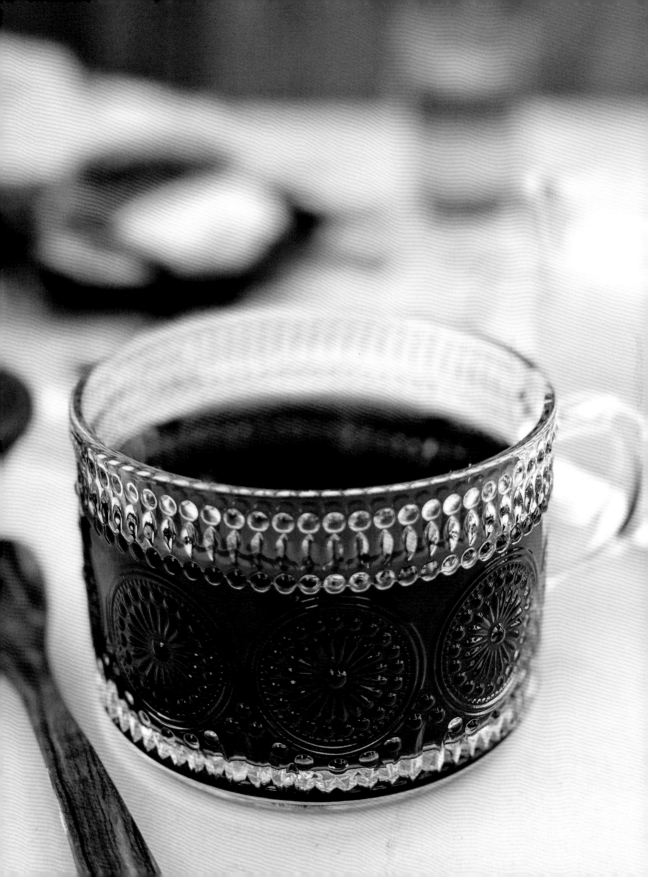

## FEEL-GOOD BEVERAGES

. . . . . . . . . . . . . . . . . . . . . . . . . . . . . . . . . . . . . . .

For me, yummy beverages play a big part in feeling good. Don't you feel good with a warm mug in your hands? Especially when what's inside the mug is so delicious and nourishing? I've included these drink recipes in the breakfast chapter, but you can enjoy them as a healthful snack any time of day.

## MATCHA LATTE

SERVES 2

. . . . . . . . . . . . . . . . . . . . . . . . . . . . . . . . . . . . . . .

TO MAKE VEGETARIAN, USE VEGETARIAN PROTEIN POWDER INSTEAD OF COLLAGEN PEPTIDES.

1½ cups unsweetened coconut milk or nut milk

2 teaspoons matcha green tea powder, preferably organic Japanese (such as Jade Leaf Organic or Pique)

2 scoops collagen peptides

½ teaspoon pure vanilla extract

½ cup boiling filtered water

1 to 2 teaspoons raw honey

Sprinkle of ground cinnamon or pumpkin pie spice (optional), for garnish

In a saucepan on medium heat on the stovetop, warm the coconut milk until steaming. Transfer the milk to a blender and add the tea powder, collagen peptides, vanilla, water, and honey and pulse on high until well combined. If desired, sprinkle cinnamon or pumpkin pie spice on top. Serve immediately.

## GOLDEN MILK LATTE

SERVES 1

. . . . . . . . . . . . . . . . . . . . . . . . . . . . . . . . . . . . . . .

ENJOY WARM OR ICED; VEGETARIAN

1 cup unsweetened almond, oat, or coconut milk

½ teaspoon raw honey

½ teaspoon pure vanilla extract

¼ teaspoon ground ginger, or 1 to 2 teaspoons grated fresh ginger

¼ teaspoon ground turmeric

Sprinkle of freshly ground black pepper

One 5-inch cinnamon stick, or ⅛ teaspoon ground cinnamon

Combine the milk, honey, vanilla, ginger, turmeric, and pepper in a mug and stir for 2 minutes or use a frother for 30 seconds, until smooth. Add the cinnamon stick to serve.

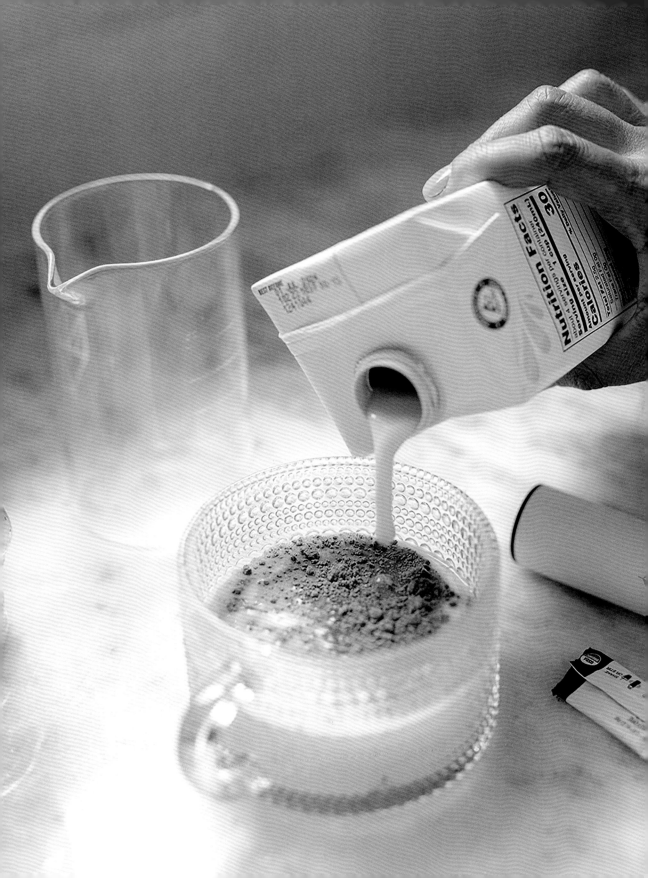

# BONE BROTH LATTE

SERVES 2

TO MAKE VEGETARIAN, SUBSTITUTE VEGETABLE BROTH FOR THE BONE BROTH AND EAT ¼ CUP NUTS OR SEEDS ON THE SIDE.

2 cups bone broth

¼ teaspoon ground ginger

Pinch of ground turmeric

Pinch of cayenne pepper

Pinch of freshly ground black pepper

1 tablespoon coconut oil

Grated zest and juice of 1 small lemon

¼ cup canned coconut cream

Himalayan pink salt, for garnish

Optional toppings: fresh herbs, chopped green onion, red pepper flakes

In a saucepan, combine the bone broth, ginger, turmeric, cayenne pepper, black pepper, coconut oil, lemon zest, and lemon juice. Warm over medium heat, stirring until combined.

Use an immersion blender to blend the coconut cream into the broth mixture. (Alternatively, transfer the mixture to a stand blender and add the coconut cream. Blend until the mixture is creamy and frothy.)

Divide the latte between two mugs. Top with pink salt and any optional toppings.

# HEALTHY HOT COCOA

SERVES 4

VEGETARIAN

4 cups milk (such as unsweetened nut, coconut, or dairy milk)

¼ cup unsweetened cacao powder

2 to 3 tablespoons raw honey

1 teaspoon pure vanilla extract

Dash of ground cinnamon (optional)

In a medium saucepan, combine the milk, cacao powder, honey, vanilla, and cinnamon (if using) and warm over medium heat, stirring constantly with a whisk. Pour into mugs and serve.

# PUMPKIN SPICE LATTE

SERVES 1

VEGETARIAN

1 freshly brewed shot of espresso or
   4 ounces extra-strong coffee

3 tablespoons pumpkin puree

⅛ teaspoon pumpkin pie spice, plus more
   for sprinkling

⅛ teaspoon pure vanilla extract

1 to 2 teaspoons maple syrup,
   or 4 to 6 drops liquid stevia

¾ cup milk (such as unsweetened nut,
   coconut, or dairy milk)

Cinnamon (optional)

In a mug, combine the espresso, pumpkin puree, pumpkin pie spice, and vanilla.

In another mug or a carafe, combine the maple syrup and milk and froth using an espresso maker or frothing stick. Pour the frothed milk on top of the espresso and sprinkle with additional pumpkin spice or cinnamon. Stir and enjoy!

# PEPPERMINT MOCHA LATTE

SERVES 1

VEGETARIAN

1 freshly brewed shot of espresso or
   4 ounces strong coffee

2 tablespoons unsweetened cacao powder

½ teaspoon pure vanilla extract

2 to 3 drops peppermint extract

2 to 3 teaspoons raw honey or pure maple
   syrup

¾ cup milk (such as unsweetened nut,
   coconut, or dairy milk)

In a mug, combine the espresso, cacao powder, vanilla, and peppermint. Add the honey and stir. In another mug or carafe, froth the milk using an espresso maker or frothing stick. Pour the frothed milk on top.

# BLUEBERRY PECAN BLENDER MUFFINS

*T*his muffin recipe could be the easiest one you've ever made, because all you do is throw most of the ingredients into the blender or food processor and then stir in the nuts and blueberries. Your kids will love these as an addition to their lunch, or maybe they'll want to have three of them for their breakfast!

**MAKES 12 MUFFINS**

2 eggs

2 egg whites

2 tablespoons coconut oil, melted

1 teaspoon pure vanilla extract

¼ cup raw honey or pure maple syrup

1 tablespoon apple cider vinegar or fresh lemon juice

2 cups almond flour

½ teaspoon baking soda

½ teaspoon Himalayan pink salt

1 cup fresh blueberries

⅔ cup chopped pecans

Preheat the oven to 350°F. Line 12 cups of a muffin tin with silicone muffin cups.

In a blender, combine the whole eggs, egg whites, coconut oil, vanilla, honey, vinegar, flour, baking soda, and salt and mix well. Gently fold in the blueberries and pecans.

Divide the batter among the muffin cups and bake until a toothpick comes out clean, about 25 minutes.

Let the muffins cool in the pan for 10 minutes before transferring to a wire rack to cool completely.

# STUFFED PEARS

*T*here's a chance this recipe will completely blow your mind. It's so simple and quick, and yet . . . the depth of flavor! If you decide to broil the pear, well, your taste buds are liable to explode. I love a slightly broiled fruit for breakfast or dessert. As you learn different techniques to incorporate more colors into your day, such as broiling colorful fruit, your hair, skin, and immune health will thank you!

**SERVES 1**

VEGETARIAN

1 medium pear

¼ cup coarsely chopped toasted pecans

1 tablespoon pepitas

¼ teaspoon ground cinnamon

1 tablespoon raw honey

Flaxseed meal, hemp seeds, or chia seeds, for sprinkling

Halve the pear lengthwise and core with a melon baller or spoon to make a well. If you'd like, you can then broil for about a minute to soften the pear, but this step is optional.

In a medium bowl, combine the pecans, pepitas, cinnamon, and honey. Fill the pear halves with the pepitas mixture. Sprinkle with flaxseed meal and eat with a spoon.

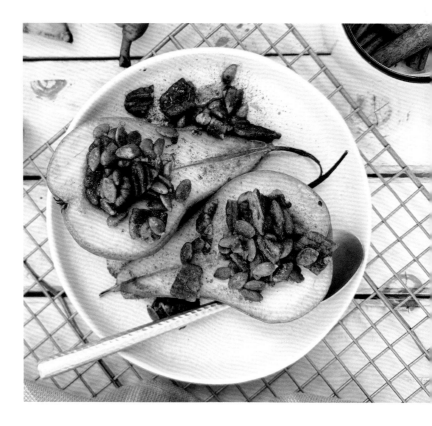

# PUMPKIN SPICE DONUTS WITH
# MAPLE ALMOND DRIZZLE

*Y*ou read that right: *donuts!* And the good news is you don't have to wait until pumpkin spice season—I mean fall—to enjoy them. You can make them year-round as long as you keep some canned pumpkin in your pantry. These donuts are moist and delicious, but user beware: it's not as easy to listen to your fullness cues here because they are so delicious! This recipe entails a little bit longer of a process than most of our other recipes, so give yourself plenty of time. If using a standard 6-donut pan, you'll need to bake two batches.

**MAKES 12 DONUTS**
. . . . . . . . . . . . . . . . . . . . . .

Coconut or avocado oil cooking spray

2 cups finely ground almond flour

¼ cup arrowroot or tapioca starch

⅔ cup coconut sugar or maple sugar

¼ cup collagen peptides

1 tablespoon pumpkin pie spice

¼ teaspoon sea salt

1 cup canned pumpkin puree

¼ cup tahini (with a drippy consistency)

2 eggs

1 teaspoon apple cider vinegar

1 teaspoon pure vanilla extract

Preheat the oven to 350°F. Generously grease the 6 wells of a donut pan with cooking spray.

In a large bowl, combine the flour, arrowroot, coconut sugar, collagen peptides, pumpkin pie spice, and salt. In a medium bowl, whisk together the pumpkin puree, tahini, eggs, vinegar, and vanilla. Pour the pumpkin puree mixture into the flour mixture and stir until combined.

Use a spoon or piping bag to divide half of the batter evenly among the 6 donut wells. Tap the pan on the counter a few times to let any air bubbles rise to the top.

Bake until the edges are just slightly browned and a toothpick comes out clean, 15 to 18 minutes.

## MAPLE ALMOND DRIZZLE

1 tablespoon coconut oil, melted

1 tablespoon natural almond butter or tahini

1½ teaspoons pure maple syrup

¼ teaspoon pumpkin pie spice, plus more for topping

Meanwhile, if desired, make the maple almond drizzle: In a small bowl or ramekin, combine the coconut oil, almond butter, maple syrup, and pumpkin pie spice. Mix into a drippy glaze.

Let the donuts cool in the pan for several minutes before popping them out to cool completely on a wire rack.

Use a spoon or fork to top each donut with the drizzle. Add another sprinkle of pumpkin pie spice.

Repeat with other half of batter to bake the second batch.

For maximum freshness, store the donuts in the fridge and reheat them in the microwave when you're ready to enjoy them. Microwave about 20 seconds if refrigerated.

# CINNAMON SPICE PROTEIN PANCAKES

*A*gain, you don't have to wait until these are seasonal to enjoy them. You can adjust the amount of cinnamon spice you're using based on your taste—and the same goes for any spices or herbs in any of our recipes. While they all provide various phytochemical benefits, spices and herbs don't impact any macros, so you're welcome to make and eat these recipes according to your taste buds.

SERVES 4 TO 6

1 large very ripe banana

1¾ cups rolled oats or gluten-free oats

1½ cups 2% milkfat cottage cheese

1 tablespoon pure vanilla extract

4 eggs

1 tablespoon flaxseed meal

1 to 2 teaspoons ground cinnamon

2½ teaspoons baking powder

Pinch of sea salt

2 teaspoons pure maple syrup (optional)

Coconut or avocado oil cooking spray

OPTIONAL MIX-INS

½ cup chopped pecans or walnuts

1 cup fresh blueberries

1 cup sliced apple

⅓ cup mini dark chocolate chips

In a blender, combine the banana, oats, cottage cheese, vanilla, eggs, flaxseed meal, cinnamon, baking powder, salt, and maple syrup (if using). Blend until the cottage cheese is smooth. If you are using any of the optional mix-ins, gently fold them into the batter.

Preheat a griddle or nonstick skillet to medium heat and lightly grease the surface with cooking spray. Ladle the batter by the ¼ cup onto the preheated griddle, evenly spacing apart the pancakes.

Cook until bubbles rise to the surface and the edges are starting to firm, 3 to 4 minutes. Flip and cook until golden brown on the second side, another 3 to 4 minutes. Repeat with the remaining batter. If needed, keep the pancakes warm in a 200°F oven while you cook the rest of the batter.

NOTE: You can double the recipe and freeze the extra pancakes in individual portions. When you're ready to serve, pop the pancake in the microwave for 15 seconds for a quick and easy breakfast during the week.

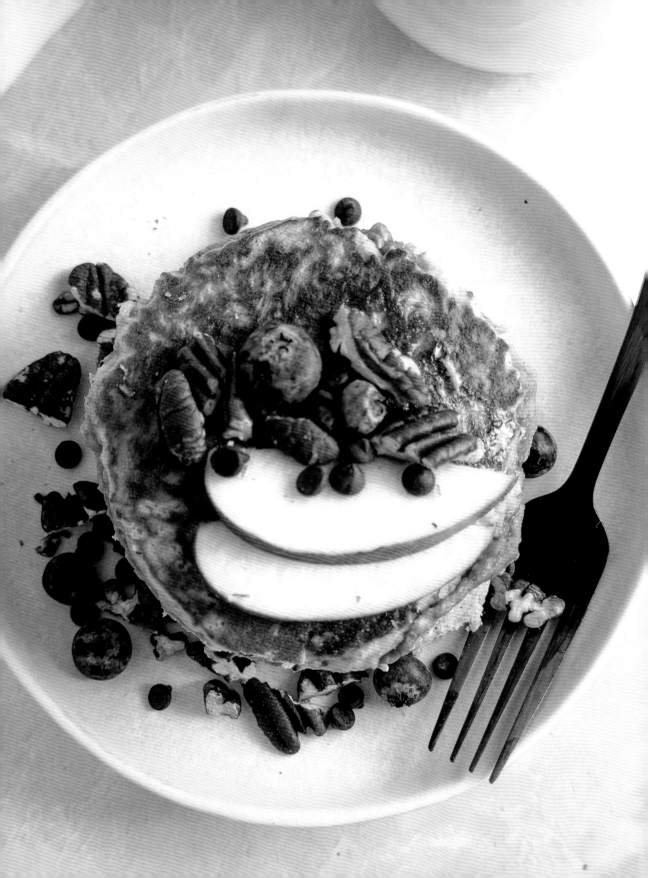

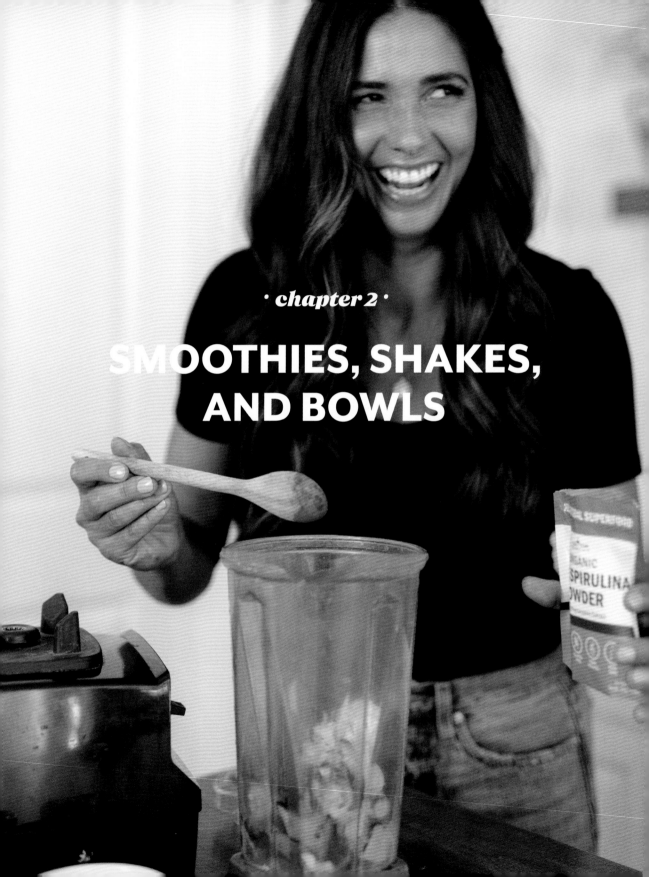

· *chapter 2* ·

# SMOOTHIES, SHAKES, AND BOWLS

. . . . . . . . . . . . . . . . . . . .

***Smoothies flood our*** bodies with nutrients. Unlike juices, which have been stripped of meaningful nutrients, smoothies contain soluble fiber, which gives your body more time to absorb all the nutrients. Instead of flying through your body like a firehose, the nutrients slowly move their way through, allowing you to digest and use the good stuff to the fullest. Another thing to love about a smoothie? It's not a salad! Not everyone craves salads—even the idea of eating salads all the time can deter people from eating healthfully. A smoothie has all the benefits of a salad and is an easy way to get more colors into your diet. I like to think of a smoothie as a salad in a cup with a hint of sweetness. And sometimes I prefer them even thicker—in a bowl and eaten with a spoon.

Before I eat, even if it's just a smoothie, I take a moment to slow down and bless my meal or take slow, purposeful breaths. This relaxes my body into a calm state that will welcome digestion and absorption. That way, none of the natural vitamins and minerals that I am going to ingest go to waste. I'll usually take thirty-five to forty-five minutes to finish a smoothie. Take your time so you can enjoy your food and your body can digest the nutrients without an anxious nervous system rushing it.

***Oh God,*** bless this smoothie to the nourishment of my whole body, mind, and spirit. Bless it to flood my body with nutrients that provide me energy that I can feel. Bless these nutrients and real food to bring healing I may need and return my body to homeostasis. These foods so rich in vitamins and minerals are such a blessing to my life. I'm thankful for them and thankful my body can utilize them. Help me to see this change in my health not as a punishment but as a privilege that I am so incredibly grateful for. We ask these blessings in your name. Amen.

Keep in mind, a smoothie is not a required part of your day or a necessary meal on top of all the others—these smoothies simply give you another option. They can serve as breakfast, lunch, dinner, or a snack.

## FREEZING SMOOTHIES SO THEY'RE READY TO GO

**METHOD 1:** Pack all the smoothie ingredients except the liquid into ziplock bags—or better yet, reusable storage bags. Then label the bags with the smoothie variation and the freeze date, and pop them in the freezer. You can keep them frozen for up to 1 month before using. When you're ready, add the frozen ingredients plus the liquid to your blender and spin your smoothie!

**METHOD 2:** Make the whole smoothie ahead of time. Blend it up, pour it into a pint-size freezer-safe jar, throw on a lid, label, and freeze. This method tastes best within a week of freezing, but you could keep the smoothie frozen for up to 1 month. Take the jar out of the freezer right when you wake up and enjoy the smoothie as your second meal of the day. Keep in mind that it will take some time to thaw, and it may need a stir to best enjoy.

# SUPER STRAWBERRY RHUBARB SMOOTHIE

*T*he best time to make this smoothie is the beginning of summer, when the strawberries are at their ripest. Usually we recommend frozen fruit for smoothies because it's fruit that has been flash-frozen right at the height of the harvest season, preserving the nutrients really well. But there is nothing better than fresh summer strawberries. Their season happens to coincide with rhubarb as well. This is not to say you can't use frozen rhubarb and strawberries, but at some point, I'd love for you to try them fresh and in season.

**MAKES 1 SMOOTHIE**
. . . . . . . . . . . . . . . . . . . . . . .
VEGETARIAN

½ frozen banana

1 cup fresh or frozen strawberries

½ cup chopped fresh or frozen rhubarb (or celery if you can't find rhubarb)

½ small beet, chopped

Handful of dark greens (such as spinach, kale, or chard)

½ teaspoon pure vanilla extract

¼ cup canned coconut cream or cream off the top of canned full-fat coconut milk

2 tablespoons chia seeds

¾ cup unsweetened coconut or nut milk

1 teaspoon maca powder (optional)

1 pitted date (optional)

Ice (optional)

Unsweetened shredded coconut (optional), for serving

In a blender, combine the banana, strawberries, rhubarb, beet, dark greens, vanilla, coconut cream, chia seeds, milk, and, if using, the maca powder, date, and ice. Blend to desired consistency. If desired, top with coconut to serve.

# KEY LIME PIE SMOOTHIE

*Y*ou can take yourself to the tropics of the Florida Keys with this sensational smoothie. It's so delicious, it may be the perfect replacement for pie. Not that I'm suggesting your pie needs to be replaced! Remember the 80/20 rule—eating well 80 to 90 percent of the time and indulging 10 to 20 percent of the time, aka living life? If you love Key lime, you will love this smoothie *and* it counts as eating well.

**MAKES 1 SMOOTHIE**
............................
VEGETARIAN

1 frozen banana

½ cup 2% plain Greek yogurt

½ teaspoon pure vanilla extract

½ teaspoon grated Key lime zest

1 tablespoon fresh Key lime juice

½ cup unsweetened milk (almond, coconut, or low-fat dairy)

1 or 2 pitted dates (optional)

In a blender, combine the banana, yogurt, vanilla, lime zest, lime juice, milk, and dates (if using) and blend to your desired consistency. If desired, rim the glass with lime zest.

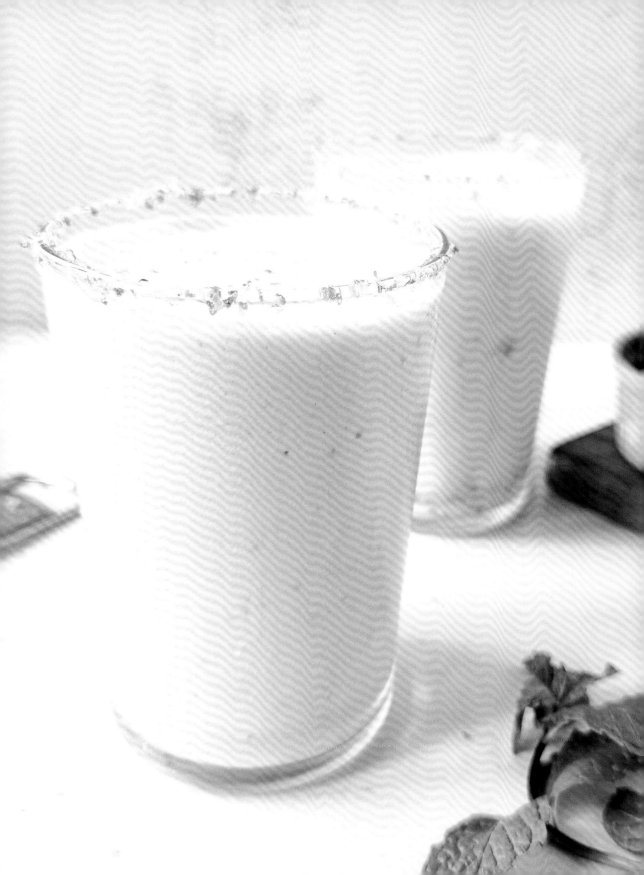

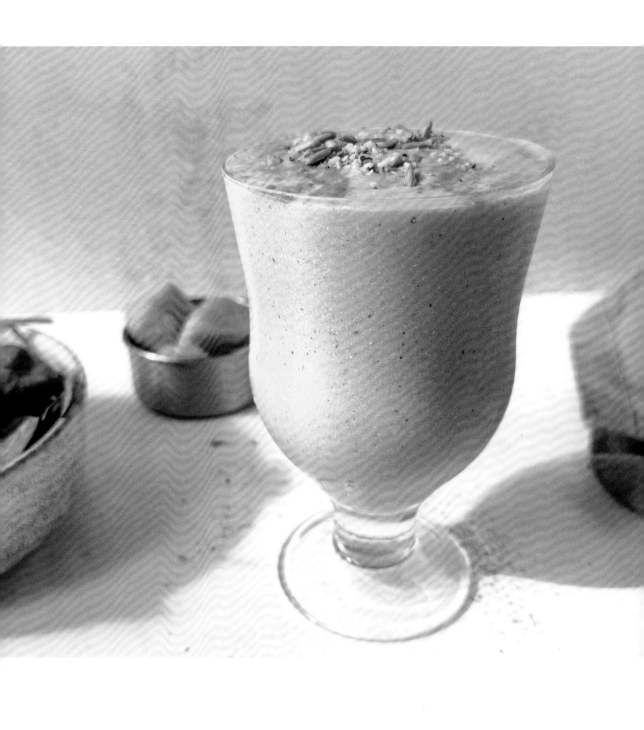

# GREEN GODDESS SMOOTHIE

*T*his smoothie will satisfy your hunger and your fiber needs—there's no doubt about that! The sweetness from the frozen mango is very subtle; if you're used to sweeter smoothies, give yourself some time with this one as the taste isn't sweet right off the bat, and it might be a slightly newer flavor and consistency for you. Our smoothies are loaded with healthy fats and protein to balance your blood sugar, so you don't need to add any additional protein—but you're welcome to add a clean (minimally processed, with natural ingredients) protein powder or collagen peptides if you feel like you need it.

**MAKES 1 SMOOTHIE**

VEGETARIAN

1 cup frozen mango chunks

Large handful of greens (such as spring mix, spinach, or collard greens)

¼ small avocado

Juice of 1 lemon

1 teaspoon ground turmeric

1 tablespoon sunflower seeds

1 tablespoon hemp seeds

½ to 1 cup unsweetened coconut or nut milk

1 teaspoon maca powder (optional)

Ice (optional)

In a blender, combine the mango, greens, avocado, lemon juice, turmeric, sunflower seeds, hemp seeds, milk, maca powder (if using), and ice (if using). Blend to your desired consistency. To serve, top with more seeds, if desired.

# BANANA NUT BREAD SMOOTHIE

$S$ome smoothies you drink from a straw, and others, like this one, you eat with a spoon. It's an experience! This smoothie is dense and filling, with the advantage that most of the ingredients are interchangeable. Don't have flax? Try chia or hemp. Don't have walnuts? Try pecans or cashews. Allspice all out? Use cinnamon and nutmeg. As long as you are balancing your macros, these recipe ingredients are adjustable. Make the recipes work for you and your lifestyle.

**MAKES 1 SMOOTHIE**

VEGETARIAN

1 medium frozen banana

½ cup cooked quinoa, or ¼ cup rolled oats or gluten-free oats

2 tablespoons walnuts

1 tablespoon flaxseed meal

Pinch of ground allspice

1 cup unsweetened coconut or nut milk

1 teaspoon ground cinnamon, plus more for sprinkling

Ice (optional)

Chopped walnuts (optional), for serving

In a blender, combine the banana, quinoa, walnuts, flaxseed meal, allspice, milk, cinnamon, and ice (if using) and blend to desired consistency. Top with a sprinkle of cinnamon and walnuts (if using).

# CITRUS GINGERBERRY SMOOTHIE

*T*his smoothie is an immune-system powerhouse, utilizing some of nature's best sources of health and wellness: berries, ginger, and lemon. When ginger is listed in these recipes, use the amount you prefer, tailoring it to your own taste. If you're new to using fresh ginger, you may want to start with a little less than is called for and then work up to the full amount as the taste grows on you. Or if you know you love ginger, feel free to add more to your liking. Ginger is well known for its properties to combat nausea, inflammation, and more, so it may be a good idea to make it a staple in your kitchen.

**MAKES 1 SMOOTHIE**
. . . . . . . . . . . . . . . . . . . . . . .
VEGETARIAN

½ frozen banana

⅓ cup fresh raspberries

½ peeled carrot, coarsely chopped, or 6 baby carrots

Small slice of fresh ginger

Grated zest and juice of 1 small or ½ medium lemon

Handful of greens (such as spring mix, spinach, or collard greens)

⅓ cup coconut kefir

2 tablespoons hemp seeds

½ teaspoon pure vanilla extract

1 scoop collagen peptides (optional)

1 teaspoon maca powder (optional)

Ice (optional)

In a blender, combine the banana, raspberries, carrot, ginger, lemon zest, lemon juice, greens, kefir, hemp seeds, vanilla, and, if using, the collagen, maca powder, and ice. Blend to your desired consistency. Add filtered water if needed.

# SWEET CHERRY VANILLA SMOOTHIE

**N**ext to wild berries, cherries are my favorite frozen fruit. Someone else pitting the cherry for me? I'll take it! Cherries are high in antioxidants and vitamin A, both of which can help with antiaging and antioxidizing, while also improving immune function.

**MAKES 1 SMOOTHIE**
. . . . . . . . . . . . . . . . . . . . . . .
VEGETARIAN

1 cup frozen cherries

¼ frozen banana

Handful of greens (such as spring mix, spinach, or collard greens)

¾ cup plain full-fat Greek yogurt

½ teaspoon pure vanilla extract

1 tablespoon flaxseed meal

¾ cup unsweetened almond milk

Ice

In a blender, combine the cherries, banana, greens, yogurt, vanilla, flaxseed meal, milk, and ice. Blend to your desired consistency. To serve, sprinkle more flaxseed meal on top, if desired.

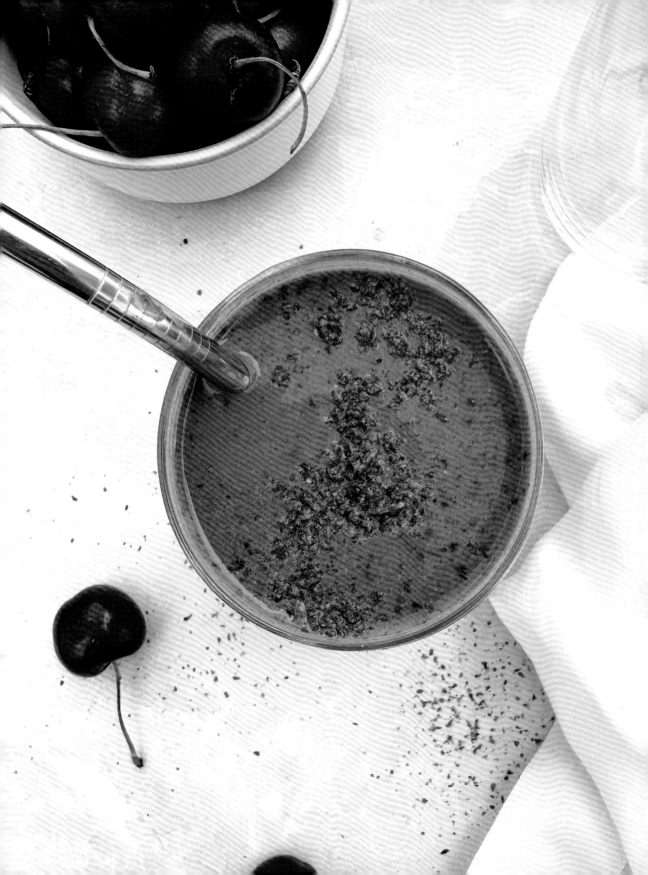

# MANGO TURMERIC TONIC

*T*his tonic can turn things around for your stiff body with just one serving. Turmeric is known to combat inflammation, which is only one of its many health benefits, but did you know that in order for turmeric to do its job well, it needs a compound called piperine to activate it? Some nutrients work better together—and in this case, the piperine from black pepper helps to magnify the potential health benefits of the curcumin in turmeric by improving the absorption of this anti-inflammatory powerhouse. And that's where the dash of black pepper in this recipe comes in!

**MAKES 1 SMOOTHIE**

VEGETARIAN

½ frozen banana

1 cup frozen mango chunks

Large handful of greens (such as spring mix, spinach, or collard greens)

1 tablespoon chia seeds

2 tablespoons natural cashew butter

½ teaspoon ground cinnamon

½ teaspoon ground turmeric

Dash of freshly ground black pepper

¾ to 1 cup unsweetened coconut or nut milk

½ teaspoon ground ginger (optional)

Ice

In a blender, combine the banana, mango, greens, chia seeds, cashew butter, cinnamon, turmeric, pepper, milk, ginger (if using), and ice. Blend to your desired consistency.

## FEEL-GOOD FAQ

· · · · · · · · · · · · · · · · · · · · · · · · · · · · · · · · · · · · · · · · · · · · · · · · · · · ·

**Should I be adding protein powder to my smoothies?**

In several recipes, I include collagen peptides as an ingredient or an optional addition. Collagen is a protein we already have in our body, and I add it to smoothies not only to increase the protein count but because it also aids our organs, including our skin, as well as our joints, bones, and muscles. A very low-processed protein powder would be another option for adding a little protein. Just make sure you choose a brand that is processed as little as possible. Many protein powders contain lots of nonfood additives for taste or texture. The final product is something very different from its original form, making it less likely our bodies will be able to use the nutrients we want from it.

# ORANGE SMOOTHIE POPS

*I* love freezing my smoothies in silicone Popsicle molds. (It's a great way to use your smoothie leftovers, too.) Making smoothie pops is especially fun with little ones in the house, and this orange smoothie pop is a for-sure winner. While I don't think hiding vegetables is necessary, smoothies are an easy way to add more veggies and colors into your family's lifestyle.

**MAKES 4 TO 6 SMOOTHIE POPS**

. . . . . . . . . . . . . . . . . . . . . . .

TO MAKE VEGETARIAN, USE VEGETARIAN PROTEIN POWDER INSTEAD OF COLLAGEN PEPTIDES.

½ cup frozen or fresh zucchini

½ cup frozen mango chunks

1 teaspoon grated orange zest

1 orange, peeled and seeded

⅓ cup shredded carrots

½ teaspoon pure vanilla extract

1 scoop collagen peptides

1 tablespoon hemp seeds

½ to 1 cup canned unsweetened coconut milk

1 tablespoon mānuka honey (optional)

1 teaspoon camu-camu powder (optional)

Ice

In a blender, combine the zucchini, mango, orange zest, orange, carrots, vanilla, collagen peptides, hemp seeds, milk, honey (if using), camu-camu (if using), and ice. Blend to your desired consistency, pour into silicone Popsicle molds, and freeze.

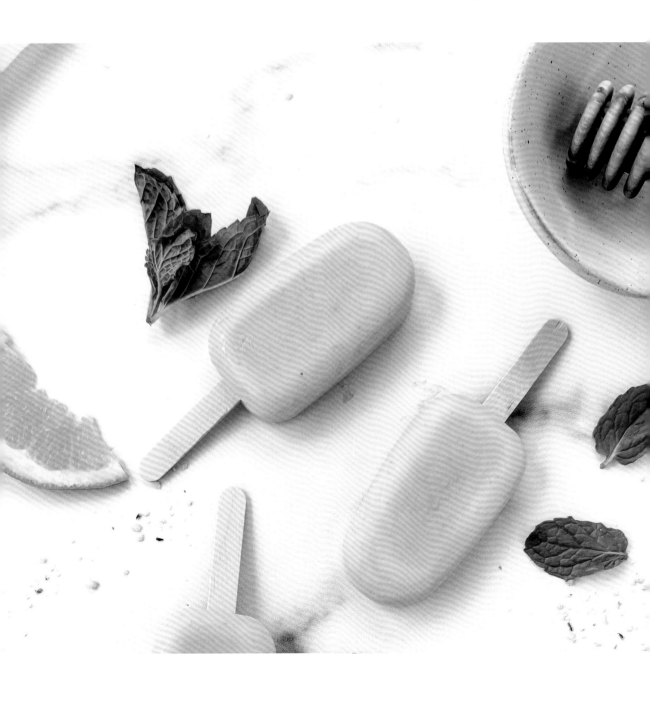

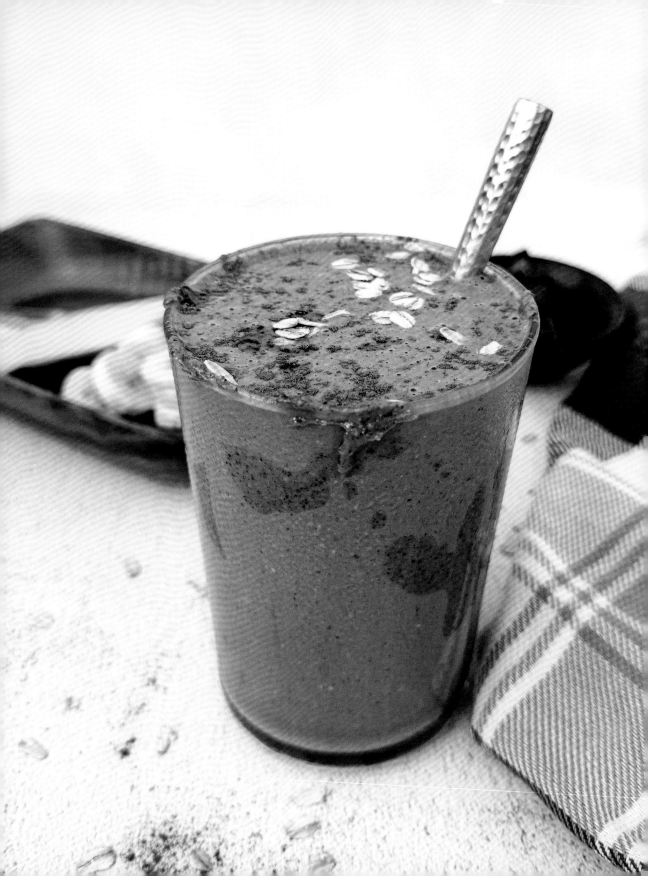

# CHOCOLATE MILKSHAKE

*T*ake note that this milkshake calls for *cacao* rather than *cocoa*. Cacao is high in the stimulant theobromine; even a small amount will deliver a great sustainable energy level, similar to caffeine but without the crash. When you start adding cacao to your daily routine, you may notice your brain feels sharper and a little less foggy than it does after that second cup of coffee. You will love this chocolate milkshake, and it will love you back!

**MAKES 1 SHAKE**

VEGETARIAN

1 frozen banana

Big handful of baby spinach

1½ tablespoons cacao powder

1 tablespoon flaxseed meal

1 tablespoon natural nut or seed butter (such as almond, peanut, cashew, or sunflower seed)

2 tablespoons rolled oats or gluten-free oats

Dash of ground cinnamon

½ teaspoon pure vanilla extract

½ to 1 cup unsweetened coconut or nut milk

1 teaspoon maca powder (optional)

1 pitted date (optional)

Ice

In a blender, combine the banana, spinach, cacao powder, flaxseed meal, nut butter, oats, cinnamon, vanilla, milk, maca powder (if using), date (if using), and ice. Blend to your desired consistency.

# TROPICAL DETOX SMOOTHIE

*T*his may not be your favorite taste right off the bat, unless you're drawn to earthier flavors. While this smoothie may be an acquired taste, it's a taste worth acquiring. It's loaded with nutrients and multiple colors, all of which offer different health benefits. The cilantro, in particular, helps cleanse the liver, delivering amazing detoxification benefits. The good news is, you don't need a huge serving of this one to experience the difference.

**MAKES 1 SMOOTHIE**

VEGETARIAN

½ cup frozen pineapple chunks

½ cup frozen mango chunks

3 to 4 leaves lacinato (Tuscan) kale, tough stems and midribs removed

Big handful of baby spinach

1 celery stalk

Handful of fresh parsley leaves

Handful of fresh cilantro leaves

Juice of 1 medium lime

1 tablespoon chia seeds

2 tablespoons hemp seeds

1 teaspoon matcha green tea powder

¾ to 1 cup unsweetened almond or coconut milk

Ice

In a blender, combine the pineapple, mango, kale, spinach, celery, parsley, cilantro, lime juice, chia seeds, hemp seeds, matcha powder, milk, and ice. Blend to your desired consistency.

# HAWAIIAN COCONUT CAKE SHAKE

When I created this shake, I was daydreaming about a delicious cake I'd had on a vacation to Maui years before. Needing a virtual vacation and a pick-me-up without the sugar, I put tropical fruit and coconut together for a dreamy combination. This shake is on the heavier side, with more healthy fat than most of our other shakes and smoothies, so you won't need to eat as much. It's perfect for those moments when you're daydreaming about a treat.

**MAKES 1 SHAKE**

VEGETARIAN

½ cup frozen pineapple
  chunks

½ cup frozen mango
  chunks

Handful of greens (such as
  spring mix, spinach, or
  collard greens)

¼ cup frozen cauliflower
  rice

¼ cup coconut cream

¼ cup walnuts (toasted for
  a deeper taste)

¼ cup rolled oats or
  gluten-free oats

¼ teaspoon cinnamon

½ teaspoon pure vanilla
  extract

½ cup unsweetened nut
  milk

1 teaspoon maca powder
  (optional)

Ice

1 teaspoon toasted
  unsweetened shredded
  coconut, for serving

In a blender, combine the pineapple, mango, greens, cauliflower rice, coconut cream, walnuts, oats, cinnamon, vanilla, milk, maca powder (if using), and ice. Blend to your desired consistency and top with toasted coconut.

**Toasting nuts and seeds** brings out their natural oils and an increased depth of flavor. To toast, preheat the oven to 350°F. Spread the nuts over a baking sheet. For whole nuts, bake 10 minutes. For chopped nuts, bake 5 minutes. Toasting coconut follows the same method, but keep an eye on it to make sure it doesn't burn.

# PUMPKIN PIE SMOOTHIE BOWL

*H*ere's a warning: This recipe tastes just like pumpkin pie, only blended up as an energizing, nutrient-dense bowl. If you haven't already been using dates in your dishes, they may become your new favorite sweetener. To me, they have a light sweetness to them, similar to maple syrup. You don't need to use a lot to taste them.

**SERVES 1**

VEGETARIAN

1 frozen banana

¼ cup canned pumpkin puree

¼ cup frozen cauliflower rice

1 or 2 pitted dates, to taste

2 tablespoons natural almond or cashew butter

1 teaspoon pumpkin pie spice

½ to ¾ cup unsweetened almond milk or other nut milk

¼ cup low-sugar clean granola (such as Purely Elizabeth) or homemade Granola (page 174)

1 tablespoon chopped toasted pecans

In a blender, combine the banana, pumpkin puree, cauliflower rice, dates, almond butter, pumpkin pie spice, and milk. Blend to your desired consistency. Pour into a bowl and top with the granola and pecans.

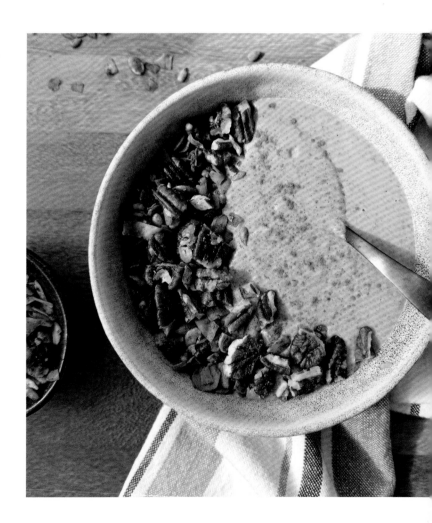

# COZY AUTUMN BOWL

*T*his bowl delivers a vibe of leaves changing, sweaters returning to your wardrobe, and fires crackling in the fireplace. If you've ever been hesitant to try squash in a smoothie, don't be. It's just as mild as regular pumpkin. You'll love the flavor combination in this bowl, so blend it up whenever you're craving that autumn vibe.

**SERVES 1**

......................

TO MAKE VEGETARIAN, USE VEGETARIAN PROTEIN POWDER INSTEAD OF COLLAGEN PEPTIDES.

1 cup cubed roasted winter squash, such as butternut, kabocha, or sugar pumpkin

½ large frozen banana

½ cup frozen cauliflower rice

1 tablespoon natural nut or seed butter, plus 1 teaspoon for drizzling

1 scoop collagen peptides

½ teaspoon pure vanilla extract

¼ teaspoon pumpkin pie spice

Dash of ground cardamom

1 dried fig, sliced

1 tablespoon pepitas

Sprinkle of hemp seeds

2 tablespoons low-sugar clean granola (such as Purely Elizabeth) or homemade Granola (page 174)

In a blender, combine the roasted squash, banana, cauliflower rice, 1 tablespoon of the nut butter, the collagen peptides, vanilla, pumpkin pie spice, and cardamom and blend to desired consistency. Transfer to a bowl and top with the fig slices, pepitas, hemp seeds, and granola. If the remaining 1 teaspoon of nut butter is not soft enough to drizzle from a spoon, microwave it for 10 seconds. Drizzle the nut butter over the bowl and serve.

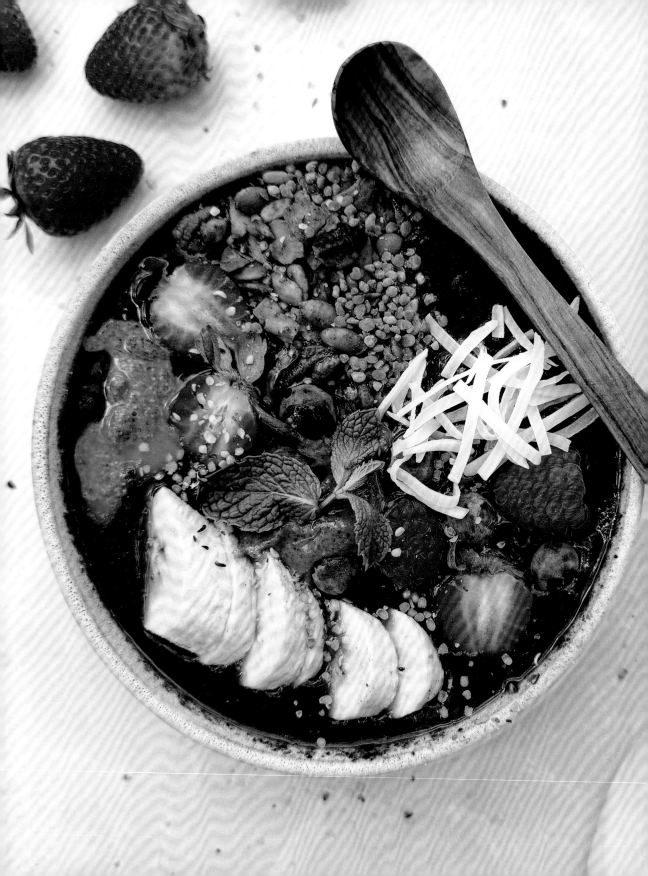

# ULTIMATE SUPERFOOD ACAI BOWL

**MAKES 1 BOWL**

**VEGETARIAN**

**ACAI BOWL**

One 3.5-ounce acai packet (found in the frozen fruit section; I like Trader Joe's or Sambazon brand)

½ cup frozen mixed berries

⅓ frozen banana

Big handful of greens (such as spring mix, spinach, or collard greens)

½ teaspoon maca powder (optional)

½ teaspoon spirulina or chlorella (optional)

1 scoop collagen peptides (optional)

**TOPPINGS**

2 tablespoons low-sugar clean granola (such as Purely Elizabeth) or homemade Granola (page 174)

1 tablespoon natural peanut or other nut/seed butter

1½ teaspoons hemp seeds

Sprinkle of unsweetened shredded coconut

⅓ banana (fresh), sliced

¼ cup fresh or thawed frozen mixed berries

1½ teaspoons bee pollen (optional)

*E*veryone I know loves an acai bowl, but generally the store-bought ones are super high in carbs without the protein and fat to balance them. When we eat carbs without enough protein and fat, we are likely to send our body into high-blood-sugar mode, which not only can cause us to store extra fat but also can desensitize our insulin altogether. You'll love this acai bowl just as much, and you won't miss the blood-sugar spike.

To make the acai bowl: In a blender, combine the acai, frozen berries, frozen banana, greens, and, if using, the maca powder, spirulina, and collagen peptides. Blend to your desired consistency.

Top the bowl: Pour into a bowl and top with the granola, peanut butter, hemp seeds, coconut, fresh banana, berries, and bee pollen (if using).

# MERMAID BOWL

*I* love to make smoothies with brilliant color, but if I'm being honest, most of my smoothies turn closer to brown because I try to fit in so many different colors at once. This is one I don't mess with, though. I love the blue spirulina, and not just for the pretty color! Spirulina is packed with several essential minerals and even has vitamin B3. It also offers many antioxidant properties, making it one of my favorite natural food colorings.

**SERVES 1**

VEGETARIAN

½ frozen banana

⅔ cup frozen blueberries

1 kiwi, peeled and diced

¼ cup fresh or frozen coconut meat or unsweetened shredded coconut

Handful of dark greens (such as spinach, kale, or chard)

2 tablespoons hemp seeds

1 teaspoon blue spirulina

½ cup almond milk

1 pitted date (optional)

Ice

Unsweetened shredded coconut (optional)

Blueberries (optional)

Kiwi, sliced (optional)

In a blender, combine the banana, blueberries, kiwi, coconut, greens, hemp seeds, spirulina, almond milk, date (if using), and ice and blend to desired consistency. Top with coconut, blueberries, and kiwi (if using).

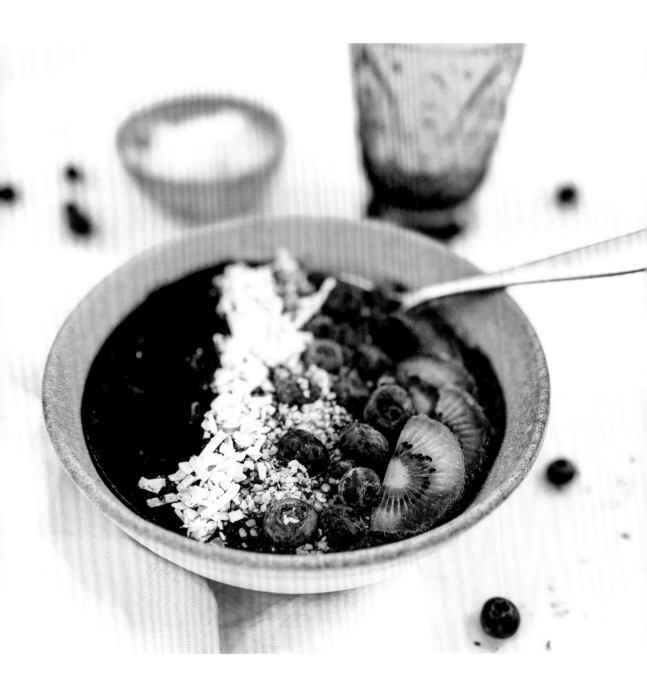

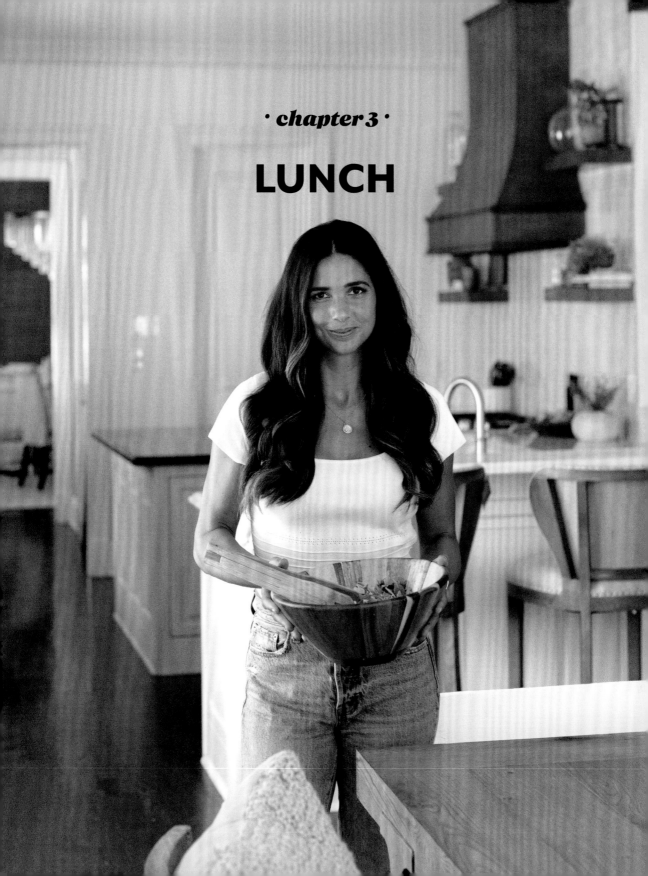

· chapter 3 ·

# LUNCH

......................

***It may not*** always feel like it, but lunch gives us an opportunity to take a breath and regulate our emotions and mood. It can serve as a break from our workload, from motherhood, from our work-from-home or corporate office. I force myself to go outside the office during lunch rather than eating at my desk.

Instead of a prayer for this time of day, I like to do a calming breathing exercise. It's an excellent way not just to step back from your busyness but also to calm your body. When we are going, going, going, and our nervous system is overactive, we experience bloating and digestive issues. Taking the time to step away, breathe, and recharge allows us to get back in touch with our spirit and body. Deep breathing can reset our parasympathetic nervous system to regulate better digestion and absorption and reduce symptoms like bloating, gas, and other digestive-related stressors.

## DIAPHRAGMATIC BREATHING EXERCISE FOR HUSHING THE RUSH AND CALMING THE BODY AND SPIRIT

Here's a simple breathing exercise that calms the nerves for better digestion. I'd suggest doing some form of this before every meal, but let's start with lunchtime. Prayer is an active form of meditation, but breathing is more inactive—not so much reflecting but just being and even receiving. This breathing exercise massages our vagus nerve, which modulates communication between our brain, heart, and gut, and allows our bodies to enter parasympathetic nervous system mode—a relaxed state that encourages better digestion and absorption and reduces symptoms like bloating, gas, and other digestive-related stressors.

**1.** Sit in a comfortable chair with your back straight but shoulders relaxed, ideally with your feet flat on the ground.

**2.** Place one hand on your heart or chest area and the other on your abdomen.

**3.** Breathe in for about five seconds—you will notice your abdomen moving outward. Hold for two seconds. Then breathe out of your mouth for seven seconds.

**4.** Repeat for ten rounds.

**NOTE:** You are not limited to ten breaths, but I'd suggest doing at least ten to start.

# LOADED "NACHOS"

SERVES 6
. . . . . . . . . . . . . . . . . . . . . . .
TO MAKE VEGETARIAN,
OMIT THE TURKEY, ADD AN
ADDITIONAL HALF OF A
15-OUNCE CAN OF BLACK
BEANS, AND USE VEGETABLE
BROTH INSTEAD OF BONE
BROTH.

1 tablespoon avocado oil

¼ onion, chopped

1 garlic clove, minced

1 tablespoon chopped
    fresh cilantro

1 pound ground organic
    turkey

1 teaspoon garlic powder

1 teaspoon ground cumin

Sea salt and freshly ground
    black pepper

One 15-ounce can organic
    black beans, drained

½ cup tomato sauce

¼ cup bone broth

24 mini multicolored bell
    peppers, halved and
    seeded

2 tablespoons sliced black
    olives

1 jalapeño chile (optional),
    sliced

FOR SERVING

3 cups cooked brown rice

Salsa

Sliced avocado (optional)

*I* personally love nachos, and watching others enjoy them is almost as satisfying as eating them myself! Typically nachos at my house are reserved for taco leftovers, but these "nachos," which use peppers instead of chips, can stand in for any meal. They're so good, filling, and nutrient-dense. They truly are loaded with colors, fiber, plenty of protein, and the perfect crunch. They would even make for great leftovers, because unlike traditional nachos, they don't get soggy when you put them in the fridge.

Preheat the oven to 400°F. Line a large sheet pan with parchment paper.

In a large skillet, heat the oil over medium heat. Add the onion, garlic, and cilantro and sauté for 1 to 2 minutes. Add the ground turkey, garlic powder, and cumin and season with salt and black pepper. Cook until the meat is completely cooked through, about 10 minutes. Add the black beans, tomato sauce, and broth, mix well, and simmer for 5 minutes, until heated through.

In the meantime, arrange the mini bell peppers in a single layer on the lined sheet pan, cut-side up.

When the turkey mixture is ready, fill each pepper with the mixture and top with olives and jalapeño (if using). Transfer to the oven and bake for 10 minutes.

Serve the peppers over the brown rice topped with salsa and avocado (if using).

# DELUXE GRILLED CHEESE

Get ready for a flavor burst. You will never look at traditional grilled cheese the same way again, with its white bread and slice of processed cheese. This healthier spin is so addictive. Like so many of the recipes in this book, you can always jazz it up even more than it already is, especially if it's with additional nonstarchy vegetables that don't affect the macro breakdown. For example, I sometimes add arugula to this sandwich to enhance the flavor and nutrition even more. Making a sustainable lifestyle plan relies on taking foods you've always loved and putting a healthy spin on them. This way you don't feel restricted. You only feel good!

**SERVES 1**
. . . . . . . . . . . . . . . . . . . . . . .
VEGETARIAN

1 tablespoon grass-fed butter or ghee

2 slices sprouted-grain or gluten-free bread

1 ounce goat cheese, at room temperature

½ cup or more peppers and onion

Handful of baby spinach

½ avocado

In a small saucepan, heat a teaspoon of ghee or grassfed butter. Add in peppers and onion and spinach and sauté for 2 to 3 minutes.

Spread the butter on one side of each slice of the bread. On the unbuttered side of one slice, spread the goat cheese. Top the goat cheese with the sautéed peppers and onion and spinach. Then top with the avocado. Place the other slice of bread on top, with the buttered side facing out.

Heat a nonstick or cast-iron skillet over medium heat. Cook the sandwich until browned and crisp on one side, 3 to 5 minutes. Carefully flip with a spatula and cook until browned on the second side, 2 to 3 minutes.

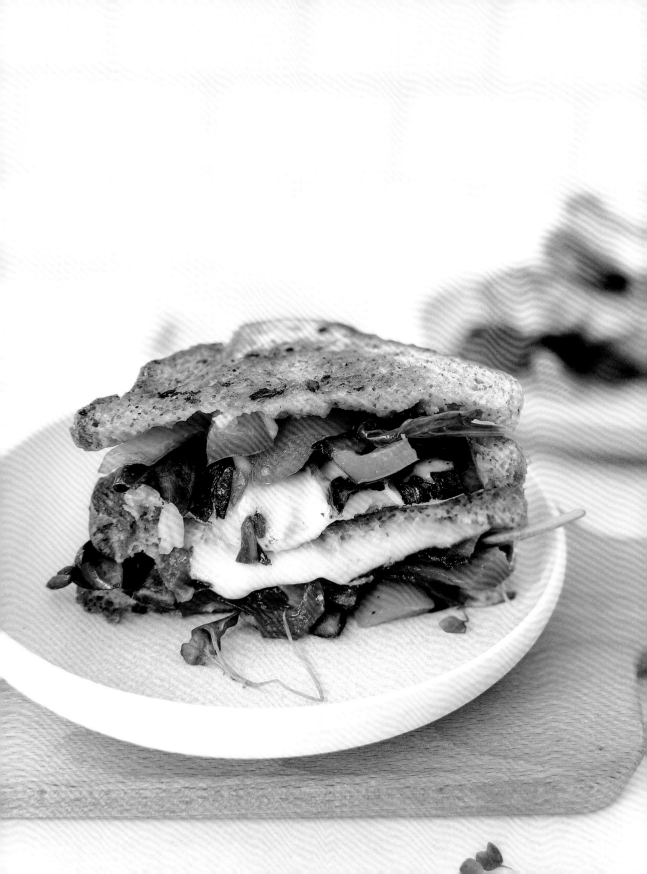

# VEGGIE PIZZA

*T*his recipe has a list of ingredients, but I genuinely encourage you to make this your own depending on what veggies you have on hand and which ones you love. You can't go wrong as long as you're incorporating plenty of protein and healthy fat, which is what the cheese offers. Feel free to add your favorite healthy meat toppings, such as turkey pepperoni, chicken, or grass-fed sausage as well.

**SERVES 6**

VEGETARIAN

8 ounces Pizza Dough (recipe follows; see Note)

¼ cup thinly sliced red onion

½ cup thinly sliced yellow summer squash and zucchini

½ cup diced unpeeled eggplant

1½ cups shredded Brussels sprouts

2 tablespoons extra-virgin olive oil

Sea salt and freshly ground black pepper

½ cup prepared basil pesto sauce (I like Trader Joe's refrigerated version)

8 ounces fresh mozzarella cheese, shredded or thinly sliced

¼ cup freshly grated Parmesan or Romano cheese

Chopped fresh basil

Make the pizza dough and let rise as directed.

Place parchment paper on a pizza pan, or if using a pizza stone, lightly grease the stone with avocado oil. If using a pizza stone, put it in the cold oven to preheat.

Preheat the oven to 450°F.

In a medium bowl, combine the onion, squash and zucchini, eggplant, Brussels sprouts, olive oil, and salt and pepper to taste. Toss to coat the veggies. Pour the veggies onto a large baking sheet or glass baking dish and spread them out evenly.

Roast for 10 minutes. Stir and continue to roast until the Brussels sprouts are browned and getting crispy, an additional 10 to 15 minutes.

Meanwhile, roll out the pizza dough in a round shape on the prepared pizza pan, or if using a pizza stone, roll out the dough on a pan, plate, or cutting board and then carefully transfer the dough to the preheated stone in the oven. Place the pan in the oven for a few minutes to prebake the crust just a bit, until it starts to rise. Remove from oven. Spread pesto sauce evenly over the dough, leaving a margin free of sauce for the crust.

Once the veggies are roasted, spread them over the pesto. Top with the mozzarella and Parmesan. Bake until the cheese is melted, bubbling, and lightly golden brown, about 10 minutes.

Sprinkle basil over the top. Let the pizza cool for just a few minutes before cutting into slices.

**NOTE:** If you'd prefer to use store-bought dough, look for a brand with the cleanest ingredients with no preservatives. Or you can use a Siete wrap tortilla instead of pizza crust.

## HOMEMADE PIZZA DOUGH

Have you ever noticed how emotionally invested you can get in cooking? Many people avoid baking because they're worried about making mistakes, but this homemade pizza dough is worth going for. It's the recipe I've found to be most successful, and your reward is that you get to have pizza afterward!

In a medium bowl, combine the yeast and warm water. Let it sit for about 5 minutes, until hydrated.

Stir in the honey, olive oil, salt, ½ cup of the flour, and, if using, the garlic powder and Italian seasoning until well mixed. Add the remaining 2 cups flour in ½-cup increments until a soft dough is formed.

On a flour-coated surface, turn out the dough and knead for about 5 minutes, until it's elastic. (Alternatively, you can use the dough hook attachment on a stand mixer.)

Place the dough in a well-oiled bowl and cover it with plastic wrap or a clean kitchen towel. Let the dough rest at room temperature for 30 minutes to 1 hour before shaping it into a pizza crust.

MAKES ONE 12-INCH CRUST
. . . . . . . . . . . . . . . . . . . . . . . .

One envelope active dry yeast (I like Hodgson Mill)

1 cup warm water (between 105° and 115°F)

2 tablespoons raw honey

2 tablespoons extra-virgin olive oil

1 teaspoon sea salt

2½ cups whole wheat or gluten-free flour

1 teaspoon garlic powder (optional)

2 teaspoons Italian seasoning (optional)

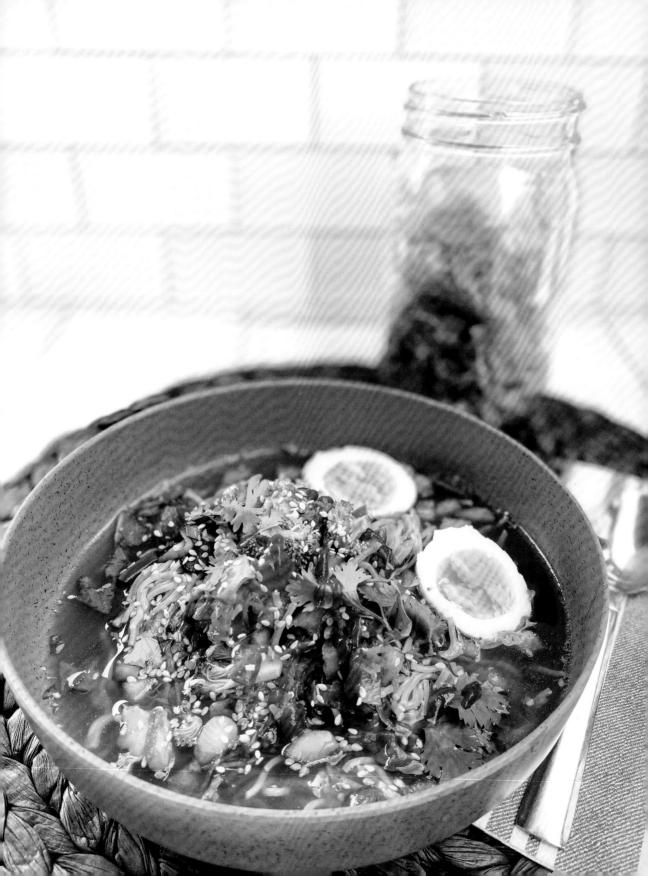

# MASON JAR RAMEN

SERVES 2
· · · · · · · · · · · · · · · · · · · · · · ·

**SAUCE**

2 teaspoons coconut
     aminos

2 teaspoons sriracha

1 teaspoon grated fresh
     ginger

1 teaspoon fish sauce

1 teaspoon toasted sesame
     oil

Pinch of sea salt and
     freshly ground black
     pepper

**SOUP**

½ cup small-diced broccoli

½ cup grated peeled
     carrots

½ cup small-diced bell
     pepper

½ cup sautéed mushrooms

1 cup chopped spinach

2 cakes uncooked brown
     rice ramen noodles
     (such as Lotus Food)

**FOR SERVING**

3 cups chicken or
     vegetable broth

Chopped fresh cilantro

Chopped green onion

Sriracha

Sesame seeds

2 soft-boiled eggs

Lime wedges

Work-lunch approved! Nobody wants to slow down during a busy day to eat, much less prepare a meal. Yet we need to eat! This ramen recipe is a no-brainer for those nonstop days. Make ahead and then heat it to eat it. It's delicious and satisfying, not to mention energy-giving. Say goodbye to those afternoon crashes, cravings, and caffeine binges because you're going to feel satisfied and invigorated with this meal.

To make the sauce: Dividing between two 1-quart widemouth mason jars, add the sauce ingredients to the jars in this order: coconut aminos, sriracha, ginger, fish sauce, sesame oil, salt, and black pepper. Mix the sauce by swirling the jars around a few times.

To add the soup ingredients: Dividing evenly between the jars, add the broccoli, carrots, bell peppers, mushrooms, and spinach. Top with the rice noodles, breaking them apart, if needed, to fit into the jars.

When ready to serve, in a saucepan, warm up the broth close to boiling. Pour 1½ cups over the contents of each jar. Screw the lid onto each jar and let it sit for 8 to 10 minutes to cook the noodles and vegetables.

Transfer the contents of each jar to a bowl and top with cilantro, green onions, sriracha, sesame seeds, and a softboiled egg. Serve with a lime wedge for squeezing.

**NOTE:** For eating at the office or on the go, add premeasured broth in a separate small mason jar to easily heat in the microwave instead of on the stove.

# CHICKEN PAD THAI

SERVES 4
........................
TO MAKE VEGETARIAN,
SUBSTITUTE VEGETABLE
BROTH FOR THE CHICKEN
BROTH. OMIT THE CHICKEN
AND ADD ONE 15-OUNCE
CAN OF CHICKPEAS OR BABY
LIMA BEANS, RINSED AND
DRAINED, INSTEAD.

1 medium spaghetti squash

1 tablespoon coconut oil

1 garlic clove, minced

1 cup shredded carrots

1 cup thinly sliced red cabbage

½ cup low-sodium chicken broth

¼ cup natural peanut or almond butter

3 tablespoons reduced-sodium tamari or coconut aminos

2 tablespoons unseasoned rice vinegar

¼ teaspoon red pepper flakes (optional)

2 cups diced cooked chicken breast

OPTIONAL TOPPINGS

Toasted sesame seeds

Chopped cashews

Chopped green onion

Fresh cilantro

*H*ere's another make-ahead-and-heat-to-enjoy meal. I don't know what it is about Asian-fare lunches, but they are so satisfying to my hunger hormones. Sometimes I feel like salads leave me wanting something else, and I find myself grabbing a handful of crackers or chips. But bowls that have a little more substantial carbs are so much more satisfying. I also love making this dish for dinner—doubling the recipe and then having amazing leftovers to eat the next day for lunch.

Preheat the oven to 400°F.

Place the whole spaghetti squash on a baking pan. Prick the skin several times with a fork. Roast in the oven for 30 to 40 minutes or until the skin is soft and slightly browned. Set aside to cool. Once it's cool, slice the squash lengthwise and scrape out the seeds with a spoon. Use a fork to scrape the cooked squash into noodles and set aside.

In a large skillet, melt the coconut oil over medium-high heat. Add the garlic, carrots, and cabbage and sauté for 3 minutes. Remove from the skillet and set aside.

To the same skillet, add the chicken broth, peanut butter, tamari, vinegar, and pepper flakes (if using). Whisk until well mixed, with a smooth consistency. Return the vegetables to the skillet along with the chicken and spaghetti squash. Toss until well coated and heated through.

Serve warm, garnished with any of the optional toppings.

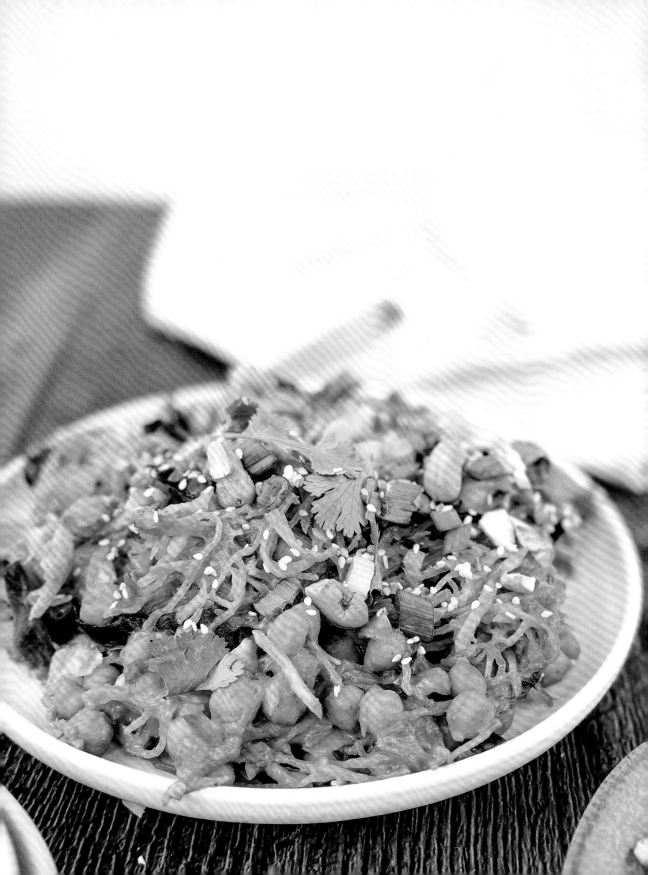

## FEEL-GOOD FAQ

. . . . . . . . . . . . . . . . . . . . . . . . . . . . . . . . . . . . . . . . . . . . .

**I get into such a lunch rut for myself and for my kids. What are some suggestions for packing a healthy lunch?**

Is there anything better than an old-fashioned Lunchable? It's one of my favorite ways to jazz up an adult lunch: crackers, meat, and cheese. Of course, we want to use the best options for these, so look for the choices that are the least processed and most nutrient-dense, such as Simple Mills crackers, Chomps grass-fed beef jerky, and raw unpasteurized cheese. Add a side of fruit and you have a great-tasting lunch box meal.

For lunches to go, I also like quinoa bowls or other power bowls (there are plenty to choose from in this chapter), mason jar salads, and a good hearty wrap or sandwich using Siete wraps or Outside the Breadbox bread.

For kids, think charcuterie board or bento box. Kids want to chat during lunch, and finger foods work well. My rule of thumb is one protein, one healthy fat (sometimes the protein and healthy fat are the same, such as nuts or cheese), one fruit, one veggie, one snack, and one treat. For lunch box treats, my kids love Dark Chocolate Zucchini Blender Muffins (page 169), homemade Granola (page 174), and energy bites (pages 230 and 231). Their lunch boxes always come home empty!

# ccn bento box guide

## veggies

cucumbers
bell peppers
carrots
celery
broccoli
cauliflower
radishes
lettuce, spinach, cabbage
snap peas
sweet potatoes
mushrooms
tomatoes

Tip: Use cutting tools
to add fun shapes to veggies
for little hands!

## protein

protein bars
full-fat yogurt pouch*
grass-fed meat stick*
chicken sausage
beans*
hummus*

hard-boiled egg*
non-preserved lunch
   meat
full-fat cottage cheese*
tuna
peas

meatballs
full-fat cheese*
nut butter*
nuts/seeds*

## treats

homemade CCN dessert
Enjoy Life cookies
UNREAL treats
SkinnyDipped almonds
Enjoy Life chocolate
YumEarth treats
Stretch Island Fruit Strips
Pure Organic fruit bars

## carbs

plantain chips
LesserEvil snacks
Simple Mills crackers
Hippeas puffs
Pirate's Booty
Nature's Bakery Fig Bars
Mary's Gone Crackers Super Seed
   Everything Crackers
pretzels
CCN muffins, waffles, pancakes
Purely Elizabeth granola
whole wheat bread or pita
wraps
tortillas
pasta, rice, quinoa
cauliflower or gluten-free pizza crust

## fruits

apples
oranges/cuties
pears
bananas
berries
grapes

mango/nectarines
raisins/unsweetened
   dried fruit
pomegranate seeds
melons
apricots

plums
avocado*
cherries
dates/figs/prunes
olives*

## favorite products

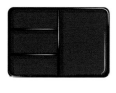
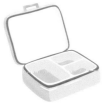

## lunch combos

**picnic**
antipasto chicken and veggie sausage skewers, sliced grapes,
LesserEvil veggie sticks, UNREAL chocolate

**mexican**
quesadilla (tortilla, cheese, sliced bell peppers), blueberries/dried
fruit, pepitas, black or pinto beans, sliced avocado

**breakfast**
CCN waffles, muffin, or pancakes, hard-boiled egg, mixed berries,
Siggi's yogurt pouch, carrot sticks

*also healthy fat

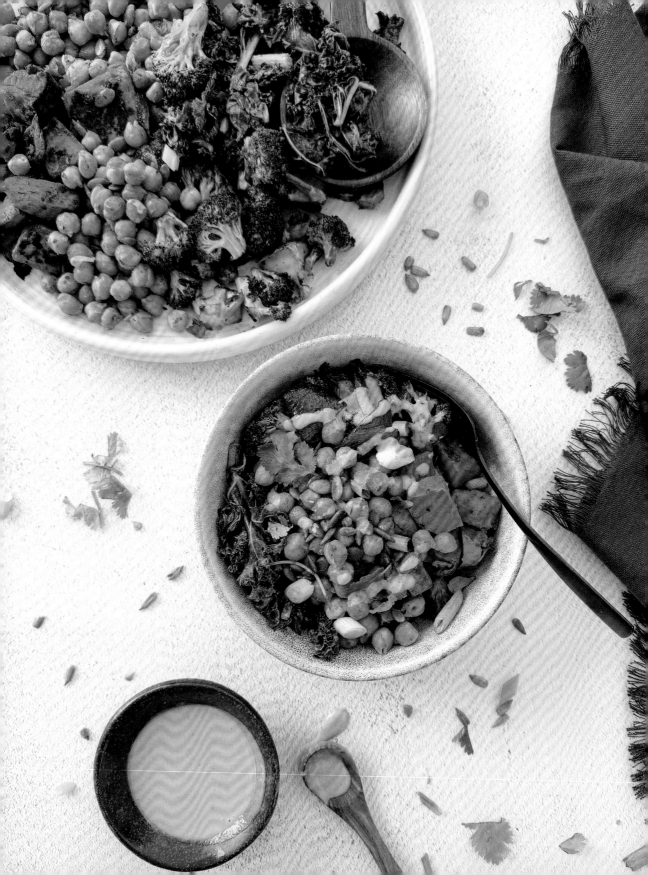

**VEGGIE MIX**

2 small sweet potatoes, scrubbed and halved

½ medium red onion, cut into wedges

2 tablespoons avocado oil

1 bunch broccoli, stems removed

Sea salt and freshly ground black pepper

2 big handfuls of kale

**CHICKPEAS**

One 15-ounce can organic chickpeas, rinsed, drained, and patted dry

1 teaspoon ground cumin

¾ teaspoon chili powder

¾ teaspoon garlic powder

½ teaspoon dried oregano

¼ teaspoon ground turmeric (optional)

Sea salt and freshly ground black pepper

1 tablespoon avocado oil

¼ cup pepitas or sunflower seeds

**TAHINI SAUCE**

¼ cup tahini

1 tablespoon maple syrup

Juice of ½ medium lemon

2 to 4 tablespoons hot water (to thin sauce)

Chopped green onion or chopped fresh cilantro (optional), for topping

# BUDDHA BOWLS WITH TANGY SAUCE

*M*ore veggies, please! I love any meal that I can get creative with to incorporate more and more veggies, especially if they're partially cooked down with a good sauté or oven roast first. Adding a healthy sauce is literally icing on the cake. Enjoy the energy you get from this power bowl—and the other bowls in this chapter—to fuel you through all your afternoon activities. The bowls are more satisfying than the average salad but just as colorful and life-giving.

Preheat the oven to 400°F.

To prepare the veggie mix: Arrange the sweet potatoes and onions on a baking sheet. Drizzle with a little of the avocado oil. Bake for 10 minutes. Remove the baking sheet from the oven, flip the sweet potatoes, and add the broccoli. Drizzle the broccoli with a bit of oil and season with salt and pepper. Return to the oven and bake for another 10 minutes. Add the kale, a little oil, and bake another 4 minutes.

Meanwhile, to cook the chickpeas: Heat a large skillet over medium heat. In a medium bowl, combine the chickpeas, cumin, chili powder, garlic powder, oregano, turmeric (if using), and salt and pepper to taste. Once the pan is hot, add the oil and sauté the chickpeas until they start to brown, about 10 minutes. Remove the skillet from the heat, add the pepitas, and stir to combine.

To prepare the tahini sauce: In a small bowl, combine the tahini, maple syrup, and lemon juice. Add enough hot water to make the mixture pourable. Set aside.

To serve, cut the sweet potatoes into bite-size pieces. Divide the sweet potatoes and the rest of the vegetables among three serving bowls. Top with the chickpeas and tahini sauce. Finish with the chopped green onion or cilantro (if using).

# CRUNCHY QUINOA BOWL

*T*he only thing more rewarding than a lunchtime power bowl is a lunchtime power bowl with a crunch. Did you know eating crunchy food can even help reduce our stress? Chewing crunchy foods reduces jaw tension, which is where a lot of our stress can build up. (Maybe that's why I find myself adding seeds or something with crunch to every salad or bowl!) In this recipe, crunchy quinoa, fresh from the oven, adds an additional step to your food prep, but you'll appreciate the inclusion. This recipe can totally be cooked ahead and stored in a jar, but I have to say it's best straight from the oven.

**SERVES 1**
. . . . . . . . . . . . . . . . . . . . .
VEGETARIAN

¾ cup uncooked quinoa

1 cup chopped romaine lettuce

½ cup shredded carrots

1 small Roma tomato, sliced

¼ cup diced cucumber

1 green onion, diced

¼ cup sunflower seeds

¼ cup diced jicama (optional)

1 hard-boiled egg (optional), sliced

**OPTIONAL DRESSING**

1 tablespoon balsamic vinegar

1 teaspoon extra-virgin olive oil

Sea salt and freshly ground black pepper

Preheat the oven to 400°F.

Meanwhile, cook the quinoa according to the package directions. Spread the cooked quinoa on a sheet pan and pat it dry with paper towels or a clean kitchen towel.

Bake the quinoa until slightly browned and crispy looking, about 20 minutes. Let it sit for a couple of minutes to cool and crisp.

In a bowl, combine the quinoa, lettuce, carrots, tomato, cucumber, green onion, sunflower seeds, and, if using, the jicama and egg.

If using the dressing: In a small bowl, whisk together the balsamic vinegar, olive oil, and salt and pepper to taste. Add to the quinoa mixture to serve.

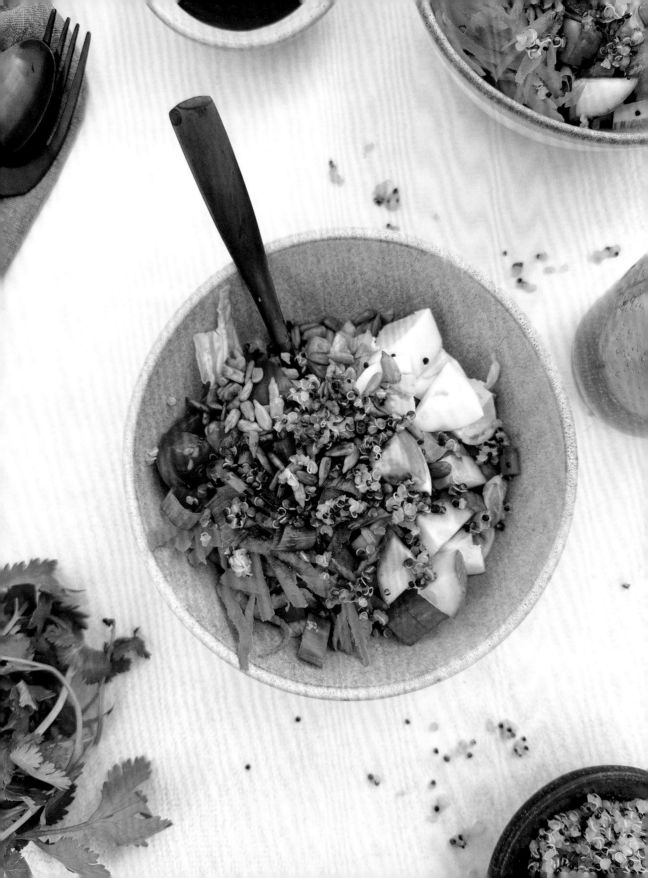

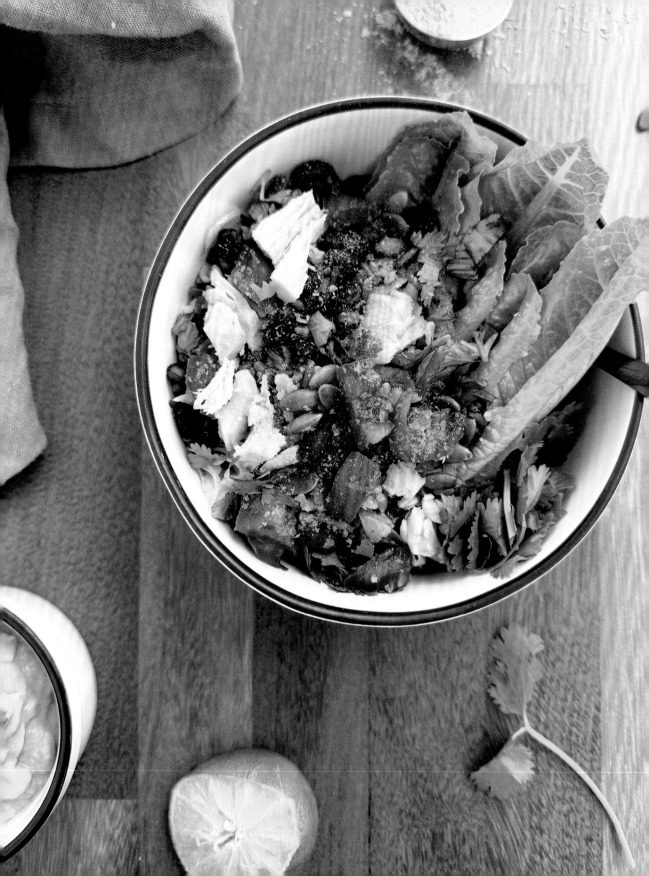

# MEXICAN CAESAR POWER BOWL

*E*veryone loves a Caesar salad—my kids especially! For me, they were always just a side and never filling enough, so I created this entrée-size version. Adding legumes and nutritional yeast is a total game changer. While I don't always need dressing on my salad, the avocado lime is to die for on this one!

**SERVES 1**

TO MAKE VEGETARIAN, OMIT THE CHICKEN AND DOUBLE THE BLACK BEANS.

2 cups romaine lettuce, chopped

½ cup chopped fresh cilantro

¼ cup canned organic black beans

1 small Roma tomato, chopped

1 to 2 tablespoons nutritional yeast, to taste

½ cup cooked wild rice

2 tablespoons pepitas, toasted

4 ounces cooked chicken breast, shredded

Avocado Lime Dressing (recipe follows)

In a bowl, combine the lettuce, cilantro, black beans, tomato, yeast, rice, pepitas, and chicken. Add the dressing to serve.

## AVOCADO LIME DRESSING

MAKES ¼ CUP

½ avocado

Juice of 1 lime, plus more as needed

1 tablespoon nutritional yeast

Sea salt and freshly ground black pepper

In a blender or food processor, combine the avocado, lime juice, yeast, and salt and pepper to taste. Blend until smooth, adding more lime juice or water if needed to thin to desired consistency.

# WARM ROASTED VEGGIE BOWL

As summer turns to fall and fall to winter, our bodies crave warming foods for a sense of comfort. Not only is this recipe a bowl of coziness, it's also another opportunity to get creative and eat more vegetables to flood our bodies with vitamins and minerals. For many people, slightly cooked vegetables are easier to digest, which makes our bodies more effective in absorbing the nutrients from these foods.

**SERVES 1**

VEGETARIAN

A big handful of kale, roughly chopped

1 teaspoon extra-virgin olive oil

½ cup cooked farro, freekeh, or other ancient whole grain, cooked in vegetable broth

1 cup steamed or roasted sugar snap peas

1 shallot, thinly sliced

1 tablespoon chopped walnuts

1 tablespoon hemp seeds

½ cup Maple-Roasted Carrots (recipe follows)

1 tablespoon Lemon Tahini Sauce (recipe follows)

In a bowl, drizzle the kale with the olive oil and massage the leaves to soften them.

In an individual salad bowl, combine the farro, kale, sugar snap peas, shallot, walnuts, hemp seeds, and carrots. Add the lemon tahini sauce to serve.

## MAPLE-ROASTED CARROTS

SERVES 4 TO 6

1½ pounds organic baby carrots

2 tablespoons avocado oil

Sea salt and freshly ground black pepper

2 tablespoons pure maple syrup

Chopped fresh parsley, for garnish

Preheat the oven to 425°F.

In a medium bowl, toss together the carrots, avocado oil, and salt and pepper to taste. Spread the carrots in an even layer on a large baking sheet.

Roast 15 minutes. Flip the carrots and roast until they are tender and caramelized, another 15 to 20 minutes. Before the last 5 minutes of cooking, drizzle the maple syrup over the carrots and toss to coat.

Garnish with the parsley to serve.

. . . . . . . . . . . . . . . . . . . . . .

Juice of 3 lemons

¼ cup water

¼ cup tahini

2 garlic cloves, grated

Dash of cayenne pepper

Sea salt and freshly ground
    black pepper

**LEMON TAHINI SAUCE**

In a blender, combine all the ingredients and blend to the desired consistency. Store in an airtight container in the refrigerator for up to 1 week.

# THREE-BEAN SALAD

SERVES 6 TO 8
. . . . . . . . . . . . . . . . . . . . . . .
VEGETARIAN

One 15-ounce can organic black beans, rinsed and drained

One 15-ounce can organic black-eyed peas, rinsed and drained

One 15-ounce can organic kidney beans, rinsed and drained

2 different-colored bell peppers, diced

1 small red onion, finely chopped

1 garlic clove, grated

¼ cup extra-virgin olive oil

¼ cup apple cider vinegar

Juice of 1 lime

Big handful of fresh cilantro or parsley, chopped

Chili powder

Sea salt and freshly ground black pepper

FOR SERVING

Lettuce or shredded cabbage

1 ounce Plantain Chips (recipe follows) or store-bought (such as Barnana or Terra)

Carrot sticks

Cucumber slices

*L*et this meal be a reminder that all Feel-Good recipes are interchangeable—this salad could be lunch or a snack or a side for a party. In fact, you will be popular if you bring this as a side to your neighborhood's next block party. Legumes offer similar nutrient profiles, with a good amount of protein, complex carbs, and fiber. But each of the three beans in this recipe offers a different variety of phytonutrients, which is why I often include several different ones in my recipes.

In a large bowl, combine the black beans, black-eyed peas, kidney beans, bell peppers, onion, garlic, olive oil, vinegar, lime juice, and cilantro. Add chili powder, salt, and black pepper to taste.

Serve over lettuce or shredded cabbage with plantain chips, carrot sticks, and cucumber slices on the side.

## PLANTAIN CHIPS

My daughters have always called these monkey chips! I think it's because the package at Trader Joe's has a monkey on it. They've become a staple in our house. Fun and easy to make, they're an amazing option for anyone who needs to follow an anti-inflammatory diet but doesn't want to give up chips.

SERVES 4
. . . . . . . . . . . . . . . . . . . . . . . . . . . . . . . . . . . . . . . . . . . .
2 large green plantains, diagonally sliced into thin "chips"

1 tablespoon coconut oil, melted

1 teaspoon sea salt

Preheat the oven to 350°F. Line a baking sheet with parchment paper.

In a small bowl, toss the plantain slices in the coconut oil. Put the slices on the baking sheet, spaced evenly apart. Sprinkle with the sea salt. Bake until lightly browned, 20 to 25 minutes, flipping halfway through the baking time.

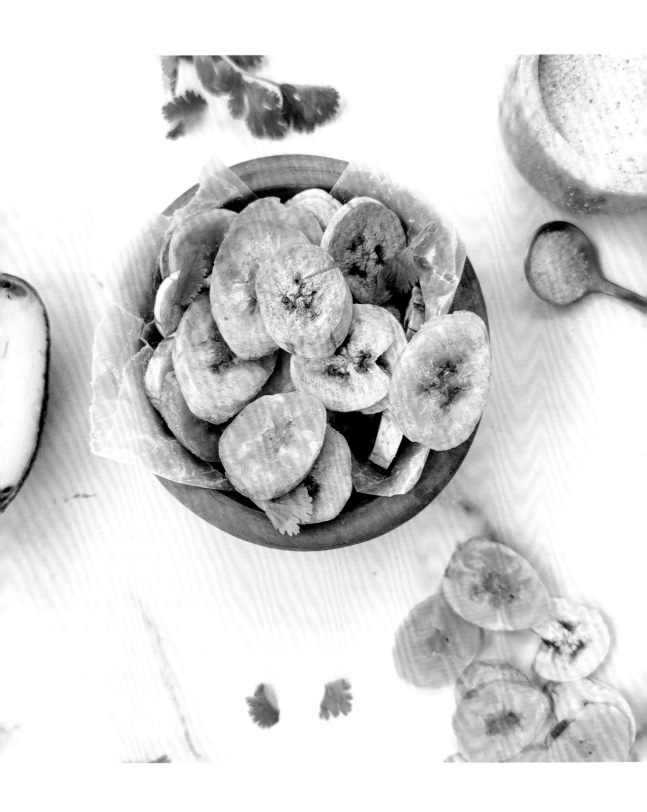

# RAINBOW NOODLE BOWL

*M*ost people don't have prep time during lunch, so all the lunch bowls in this chapter are designed to be made ahead of time. They can even be prepped for the entire week and separated into glass storage containers. Be sure to store the dressing separately and add it when you're ready to eat. (By the way, if you still have plastic food storage containers, now is a great time to make the switch to glass or another nontoxic food storage option.)

**SERVES 1**

VEGETARIAN

1 baby cucumber, sliced

1 red bell pepper, thinly sliced

1 large carrot, spiralized

1 medium golden beet, spiralized

1 large broccoli stem, spiralized

½ cup cooked quinoa

½ cup canned organic chickpeas

2 to 3 tablespoons Carrot Ginger Dressing (recipe follows), to taste

1 tablespoon chopped cashews or peanuts

Toasted sesame seeds

Small handful of fresh parsley, chopped

Red pepper flakes

Sea salt and freshly ground black pepper

In a bowl, combine the cucumber, bell pepper, carrot, beet, broccoli, quinoa, and chickpeas. Add the dressing and toss. Top with the cashews, sesame seeds, and parsley. Season to taste with pepper flakes, salt, and black pepper.

**CARROT GINGER DRESSING**

MAKES ¾ CUP

1 medium carrot, peeled and grated

1-inch slice fresh ginger, grated

¼ cup extra-virgin olive oil

¼ cup unseasoned rice vinegar

2 tablespoons raw honey

2 tablespoons coconut aminos

1 teaspoon toasted sesame oil

Sea salt and freshly ground black pepper

In a blender or food processor, combine all the ingredients. Pulse until smooth, 1 to 2 minutes. Store in an airtight container in the refrigerator for up to 1 week.

# SUPER DETOX SALAD

*T*his salad is addictive. But even though it's so good and satiating, it's nearly impossible to eat too much of it because the fiber content is so high that your body feels full faster. It might look like a side salad in size, but because of the carbs from the oranges and the fat and protein from the sunflower seeds and dressing, it will actually feel like a full meal.

**SERVES 1**

VEGETARIAN

1 cup arugula

¼ medium fennel bulb, quartered lengthwise and very thinly sliced

3 radishes, thinly sliced or diced

Radish leaves from 3 radishes, chopped

¼ red onion, thinly sliced

2 fresh mandarin oranges, peeled and sectioned

1 tablespoon sunflower seeds

OPTIONAL DRESSING

1 tablespoon extra-virgin olive oil

1 tablespoon fresh lemon juice

1 tablespoon chopped fresh mint

Sea salt and freshly ground black pepper

In a bowl, combine the arugula, fennel, radishes, radish leaves, onion, orange sections, and sunflower seeds.

If using the dressing, in a small bowl, whisk together the olive oil, lemon juice, mint, and salt and pepper to taste. Add to the salad and toss.

**FEEL-GOOD STORY**

. . . . . . . . . . . . . . . . . . . . . . . . . . . . . . . . . . . . . . . . . . . . . . . . . . .

## *Lindsay*

Doctors told Lindsay there was nothing she could do to improve her Lyme disease other than follow their medical protocol. But they told her it could take years for the protocol to show results, and it might not ever heal her body. Lindsay was miserable. She felt like she was losing hope of ever regaining her health and energy. She's the mother of three kiddos and had always been super active and a high achiever. She wouldn't accept her prognosis.

Lindsay knew that food could play a huge role in her healing. She understood that if she were absorbing nutrients better and could heal her gut, then she could start feeling better faster. All she wanted was to feel an inkling of her old self return.

At the time, I spent a lot of time engaging with moms like Lindsay. The early years of motherhood can be physically and mentally exhausting, so I wanted to teach them how to feel better and give themselves the energy to be present in the moment. I would visit MOPS (Mothers of Preschoolers) groups, giving talks about the food we eat and how even small changes in our diet can make a huge difference.

One day, I was giving a presentation to Lindsay's MOPS group. As she listened to what I had to say, she knew that God had placed this nutritionist at her meeting for a reason, and she wasn't going to let the opportunity pass her by.

She jumped in to one of the CCN programs. As she began eating real food that was macro balanced, colorful, and not overly restrictive, she started to regain a little hope and, even better, a little energy. The new energy helped her think more clearly. She visited other doctors with a more integrative approach to her Lyme disease, and while she knew she still needed to follow the standard medical approach, she also knew she was going to feel better faster than they'd originally told her. She realized that half the battle was just getting the energy she needed to make decisions.

Lindsay was able to beat the disease in way less time than the doctors had suggested, and she is now completely Lyme free! Not in remission—but absolutely free of the disease. She felt whole again and even started working in a service-oriented job to help young mothers thrive in their early stage of motherhood. She never imagined feeling good enough to serve others on that level.

Lindsay is one of a kind and totally inspiring, but all of this change started with food and fueling her body with the Feel-Good approach. Feeling good and having more energy helped her heal her own body, better her life, and be her true self. How's that for empowering?

# WALNUT BEET SALAD

*F*un fact: Beets are rich in nitrates, which convert to nitric acid in the body. Nitric acid is a compound that can relax blood vessels, which helps drive oxygen-rich blood. This improves circulation, among other things! I learned this because I personally struggled with varicose veins during pregnancy and needed a natural way to calm my veins and treat the pain. Beets and beet extract helped a lot. I used to think I hated beets, but when I realized what they could do for my body, I began loving them and looking for more ways to incorporate them into my meals. I love them any which way now, but sometimes I have a huge craving for pickled beets, so I keep jars of them on hand. They're fine to swap in for the steamed or roasted beet in this recipe.

SERVES 1
......................
VEGETARIAN

1 tablespoon hemp seeds

¼ avocado, chopped or sliced

1 cup shredded Brussels sprouts

½ cup shredded red cabbage

1 steamed or roasted baby beet, chopped or julienned

1 tablespoon golden raisins

¼ cup walnuts, toasted

½ cup canned organic chickpeas

1 to 2 tablespoons Maple Dijon Dressing (recipe follows)

Sprinkle the hemp seeds over the avocado. In a bowl, combine the Brussels sprouts, cabbage, beet, raisins, walnuts, chickpeas, avocado with hemp seeds, and dressing. Toss to combine.

## MAPLE DIJON DRESSING

MAKES ABOUT ¾ CUP
...................................................

¼ cup apple cider vinegar

¼ cup extra-virgin olive oil

1 tablespoon Dijon mustard

1 tablespoon pure maple syrup

Sea salt and freshly ground black pepper

In a small bowl, combine the vinegar, olive oil, mustard, maple syrup, and salt and pepper to taste and whisk to combine.

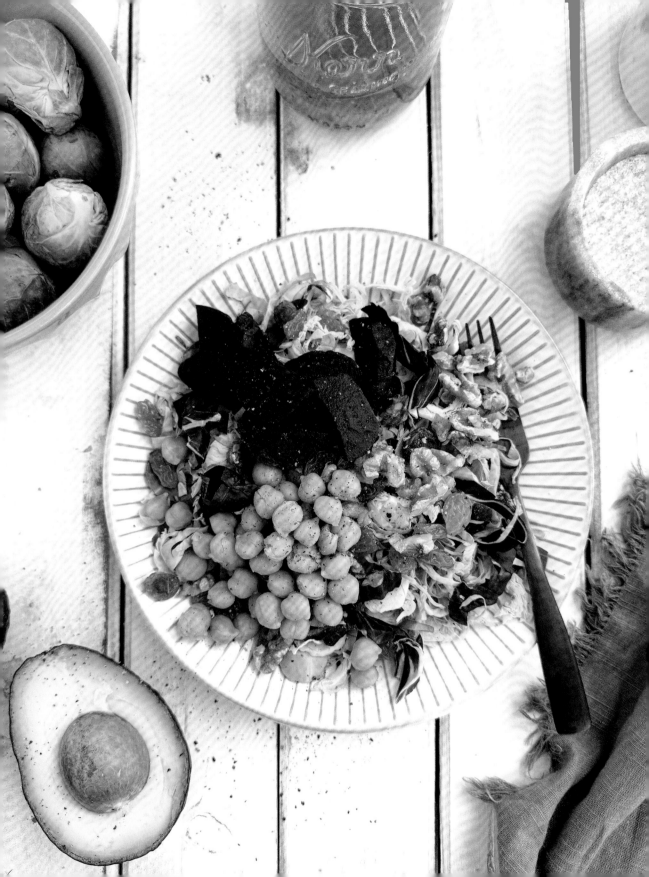

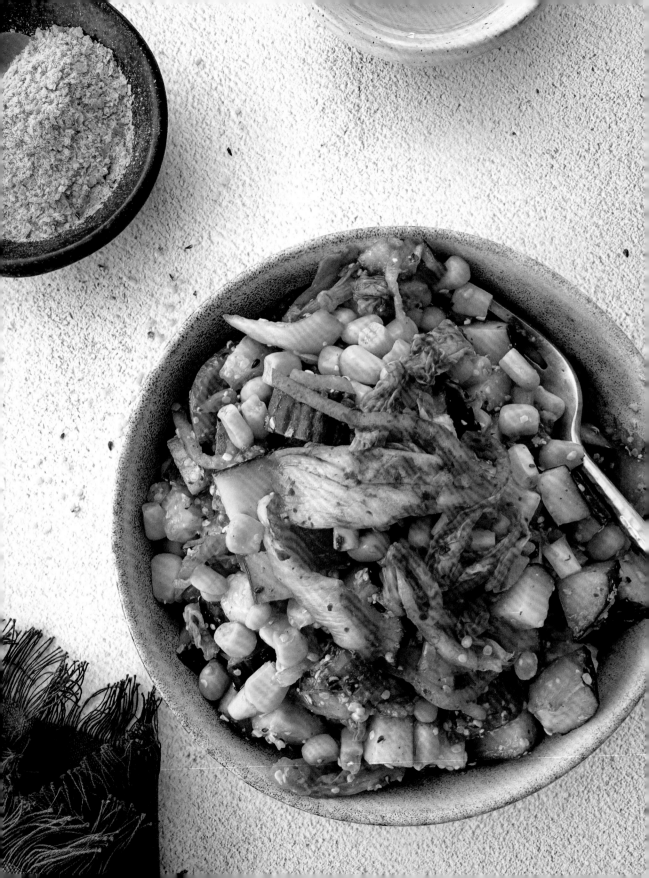

# FERMENTED CUCUMBER SALAD

*I* always loved pickles and sauerkraut as a kid, but when I grew up, I realized how many other foods you could eat pickled or fermented. Essentially, pickling/fermenting is a way to keep and store foods without using harmful additives. It also brings out a fun, alternative flavor while not only preserving the nutrients but adding even more. Fermented foods improve the microbiome colonies living in our guts. They can even help improve the intestinal lining for better nutrient absorption and bioavailability of the nutrients we're eating. In this recipe, the fermentation comes with the sauerkraut. If you think you're not a fan of sauerkraut, please give this recipe a try. I think it might change your mind!

**SERVES 1**

VEGETARIAN

½ cup sauerkraut or kimchi

1 medium cucumber, sliced or chopped

1 medium tomato, diced

¼ cup diced red onion

½ cup fresh or frozen corn kernels

1 tablespoon extra-virgin olive oil

Sea salt and freshly ground black pepper

2 tablespoons nutritional yeast

Sprinkle of hemp seeds

In a bowl, combine the sauerkraut, cucumber, tomato, onion, corn, olive oil, salt and pepper to taste, yeast, and hemp seeds. Toss to combine.

# CRUCIFEROUS CRUNCH SALAD

*I*'ve been enjoying this salad for more than a decade now, making it one of my most tried-and-true recipes. It's so satisfying and crunchy, and you can multiply it to create a big crowd-pleaser at parties. If you have digestive issues, though, it may be best for you to slightly steam the veggies first before tossing them with the dressing. Cruciferous vegetables contain a fiber called cellulose, which can be difficult to digest for some people. If this is you, you don't have to restrict these superfoods; you simply need to cook them a little first.

**SERVES 1**

VEGETARIAN

½ cup canned organic chickpeas, or 4 ounces cooked and shredded chicken breast (or 2 ounces of each)

⅓ cup finely chopped broccoli

⅓ cup finely chopped cauliflower

1 medium carrot, chopped or shredded

½ cup chopped or shredded green and red cabbage

Chopped red bell pepper (optional)

Chopped green onion (optional)

1 to 2 tablespoons Thai Peanut Dressing (recipe follows)

1 tablespoon chopped cashews or peanuts

Sprinkle of hemp hearts

In a bowl, combine the chickpeas, broccoli, cauliflower, carrot, cabbage, and, if using, the bell pepper and green onion. Toss with the dressing. Top with cashews and hemp hearts.

## THAI PEANUT DRESSING

MAKES 1 CUP

Thumb-size piece fresh ginger, grated

3 garlic cloves, grated

⅓ cup unseasoned rice vinegar

¼ cup creamy natural peanut butter

1 tablespoon raw honey

1 tablespoon coconut aminos

½ teaspoon sriracha or preferred hot sauce

2 teaspoons toasted sesame oil

2 tablespoons water

In a blender, combine the ginger, garlic, vinegar, peanut butter, honey, coconut aminos, sriracha, sesame oil, and water. Blend to your desired consistency.

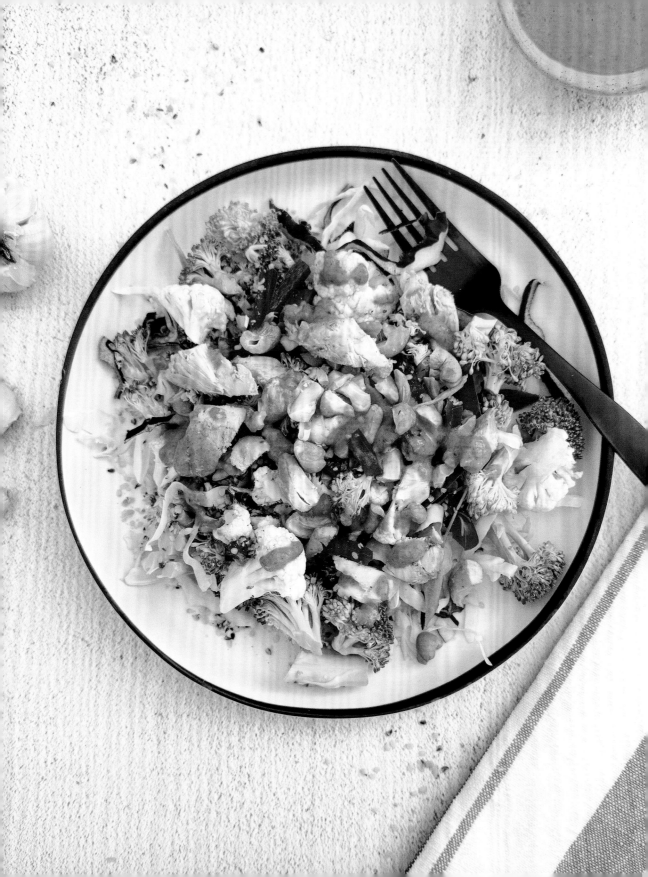

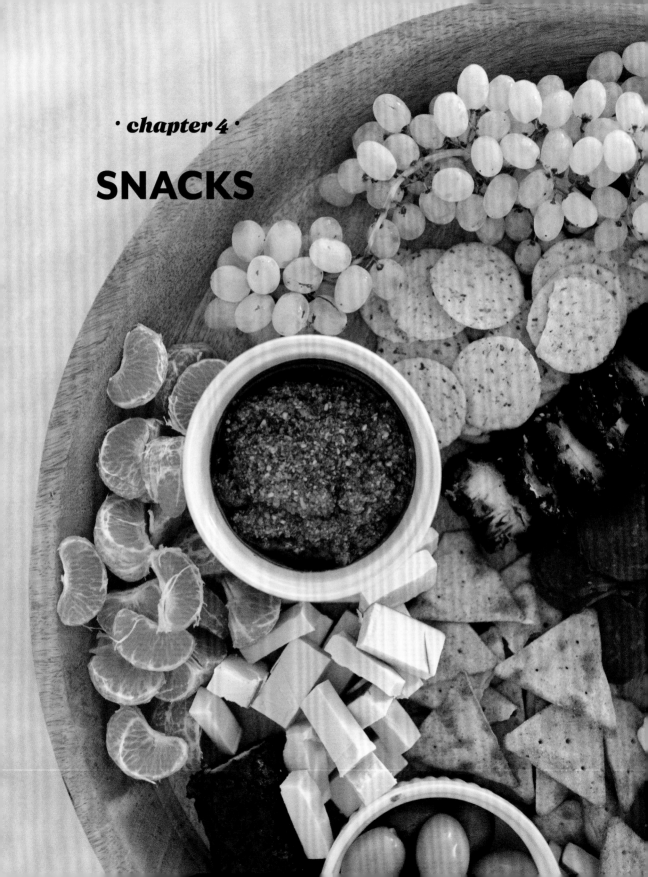

· *chapter 4* ·

# SNACKS

. . . . . . . . . . . . . . . . . . . .

**Here is our** opportunity to flow instead of fade! In the afternoon, as we transition from working back to being mom, a fiber- and nutrient-rich snack is a great alternative to letting ourselves sink into a caffeine and sugar rage. When we eat more frequently (and healthfully), we keep our glucose level stable.

These snacks pack a punch and are in the same caloric range as a meal. If you've already had a smoothie or snack in addition to meals, you probably wouldn't need an afternoon snack unless your energy needs are higher because of a change in activity. For instance, heavy weight training can really impact your appetite, and you don't need to go hungry because of it. If you need a quick bite but not a full-size snack, my favorite go-tos are trail mix, 6 ounces of Greek yogurt with fruit, walnuts and granola, nut butter and toast, cottage cheese and pretzels, energy bites, or just fruit and nuts.

I'll be honest—I don't *always* remember to say a blessing before my snacks, but when I have a moment in the middle of the afternoon to stop what I'm doing and have a quick bite, I like to reflect on my gratitude for the nourishing food and pray that it's used well in my body. When I do take the time to do this, I notice how much more I slow down, savor each bite of food, and calm my body and spirit. It's re-energizing and nourishing in every way.

**Bless this** snack to give me the energy I need to push forward in my day and not rely on sugar, caffeine, or unnecessary pick-me-ups. Bless the food to nourish my mind, body, and spirit and bridge the gap between lunch and dinner.

Reflect on your hunger and satiety cues here and sit in gratitude for the hormone system that provides these messages to the brain.

**I'm thankful** for the hunger cues that remind me that my body is low on energy supply.

I'm thankful for fullness cues to let my brain know I'm satisfied with the energy from the food I just provided my body.

I'm thankful for healthy hormones that allow glucose to enter my cells, my brain, and my liver to provide energy.

I'm thankful for a body that can utilize nutrition from the smallest cell to the largest organ in my body. At any given moment, hundreds of systems are operating on full, and I feel good when I provide myself the energy for these processes.

Amen.

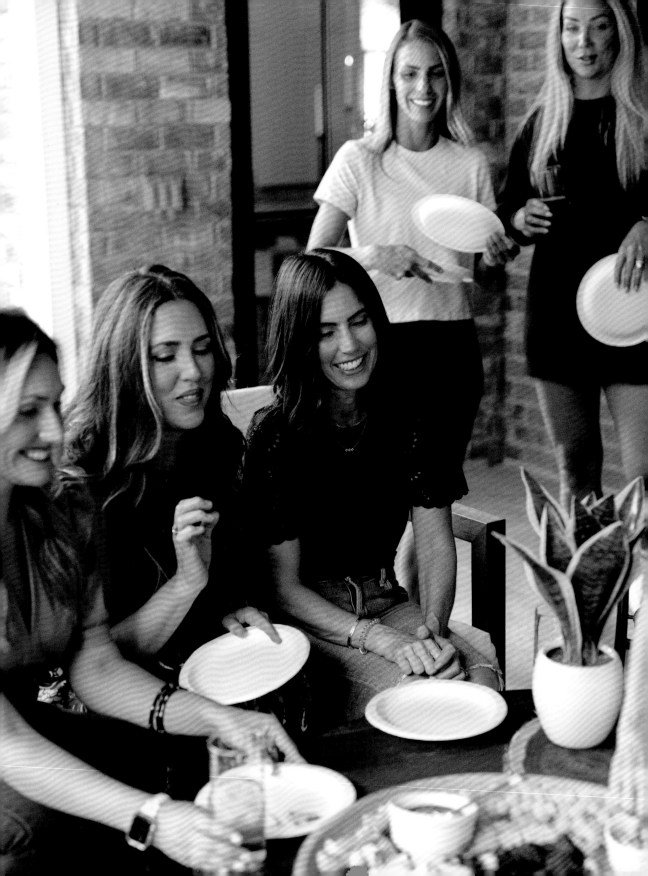

# GARLIC HUMMUS

One of the easiest snacks I keep on hand for me and my kiddos is hummus. It's as much a staple at our house as eggs, and we do not like to run out! It's great with crackers, bread, pretzels, and veggies, of course. I like to top my salads with hummus. Given all the fiber, minerals, and B vitamins it contains, it keeps me full longer. I consider it one of my personal superfoods because it provides the healthy fat and protein our bodies need, and I inevitably pair it with lots of colorful veggies.

**MAKES ABOUT 1 CUP**

**VEGETARIAN**

2 heads garlic

2 tablespoons extra-virgin olive oil

One 15-ounce can organic chickpeas, rinsed and drained

Juice of 2 medium lemons

3 tablespoons tahini

¼ cup nutritional yeast

Sliced peppers, carrots, cucumber, celery, or almond-based crackers, for serving

Preheat the oven to 350°F.

Peel away the papery outer skin of the garlic heads. Cut off the tops, about ½ inch, to expose the cloves. Place on a sheet of foil and drizzle with the olive oil. Crimp the foil closed.

Roast the garlic for 1 hour.

Let the garlic cool fully before handling, then squeeze the roasted garlic cloves out of the skin and into a blender. Add the chickpeas, lemon juice, tahini, and yeast. Blend until smooth.

Serve with the veggie slices or crackers. Store in an airtight container in the fridge for 7 to 10 days. This stores well in the freezer, too.

# BROWNIE FRUIT DIP

*L*ike hummus but a treat. I dare you to not eat this while you're making it. You might lick the spoon so many times, you'll be full before it's finished. If you're put off by the idea of combining kidney beans with chocolate, I promise you won't even taste them and you'll think you're eating brownie batter. If you make it to the end of the prep without eating it all, this dip is incredible paired with fruit. Apples and bananas are my favorite pairings, but if you happen to have gluten-free graham crackers lying around, you'll love the indulgent combination.

**MAKES ABOUT 1 CUP**
.............................
VEGETARIAN

One 15-ounce can organic kidney beans, rinsed and drained

⅓ cup cacao powder (or more or less, depending on how dark you'd like the color)

2 tablespoons natural almond or other nut or seed butter

1 teaspoon pure vanilla extract

¼ cup raw honey or pure maple syrup

½ teaspoon Himalayan pink salt

2 to 4 tablespoons unsweetened cashew milk

OPTIONAL TOPPINGS

Mini dark chocolate chips

Chopped nuts

Dye-free sprinkles

In a food processor or blender, combine the kidney beans, cacao powder, almond butter, vanilla, honey, salt, and 2 table-spoons of the cashew milk. Pulse until smooth, adding more cashew milk if needed. Serve with toppings (if using).

## FEEL-GOOD FAQ

**I have a desk job and sometimes I realize it's been hours since I moved! How can I incorporate some healthy movement into my workday?**

I love a good wall sit! Sit with your back against the wall and your hands in your lap. Start by holding it for one minute, or even thirty seconds if a minute is too long. Then, every time you try again, aim to add another thirty seconds to your clock. To take that a level further, roll your back up and down the wall, engaging your glute and leg muscles.

If you have stairs close by, walking up and down is another quick way to get some movement in and your heart rate going. You can grab hand weights or even water bottles and do some walking lunges across the floor or down a hallway. I work from home and do these a lot during long workdays when I don't have time for an actual deliberate workout. Finally, a fifteen- to twenty-minute walk outside is always a good option—good for the body and mind. Our bodies were never meant to be so sedentary, and it's time to get back to our instinct to move!

# PESTO DIP WITH CRACKERS

*B*asil, like other herbs, has some pretty amazing properties. It contains antioxidants, it helps manage blood pressure and cholesterol, and it combats pathogens and inflammation. I love growing it in my kitchen, for its benefits of course, but mostly so I can have pesto anytime I want! This pesto dip also works as a sauce or topping. It's versatile, with great flavor. You're going to love the pine nuts, but if you don't have pine nuts, I'd recommend swapping in walnuts for a similar taste. And you may want to double or triple the cracker recipe. These crackers don't last long around my house. They also don't store all that well, so keep in mind to make what you plan on eating within a day or so. If you end up with leftovers, store them with the lid loosely placed on top, not tightly. Otherwise they may get soggy. If you can't do nuts, you could swap the almond flour for tiger nut flour or a basic gluten-free flour blend.

**MAKES ABOUT 1½ CUPS**
.........................

VEGETARIAN WITHOUT THE CRACKERS

½ cup pine nuts, lightly toasted

½ cup hemp seeds

2 cups packed fresh basil leaves

3 garlic cloves, peeled but whole

1 tablespoon raw honey or pure maple syrup

Juice of 1 medium lemon

¼ teaspoon sea salt

Pinch of freshly ground black pepper

¼ to ½ cup extra-virgin olive oil

Homemade Crackers (recipe follows), for serving

In a food processor or blender, combine the pine nuts, hemp seeds, basil, garlic, honey, lemon juice, salt, and pepper. While the processor is running, slowly drizzle in just enough olive oil to create a thick paste. Serve with the crackers.

## HOMEMADE CRACKERS

**MAKES ABOUT 24 CRACKERS**
.............................................................

1¾ cups almond flour

½ teaspoon sea salt, plus more for topping

2 tablespoons finely chopped fresh rosemary

1 tablespoon extra-virgin olive oil

1 egg

Preheat the oven to 350°F.

In a medium bowl, combine the almond flour, ½ teaspoon of the salt, and the rosemary. In a separate medium bowl, whisk together the olive oil and egg. Stir the egg mixture into the flour mixture until thoroughly combined.

*(continues on page 156)*

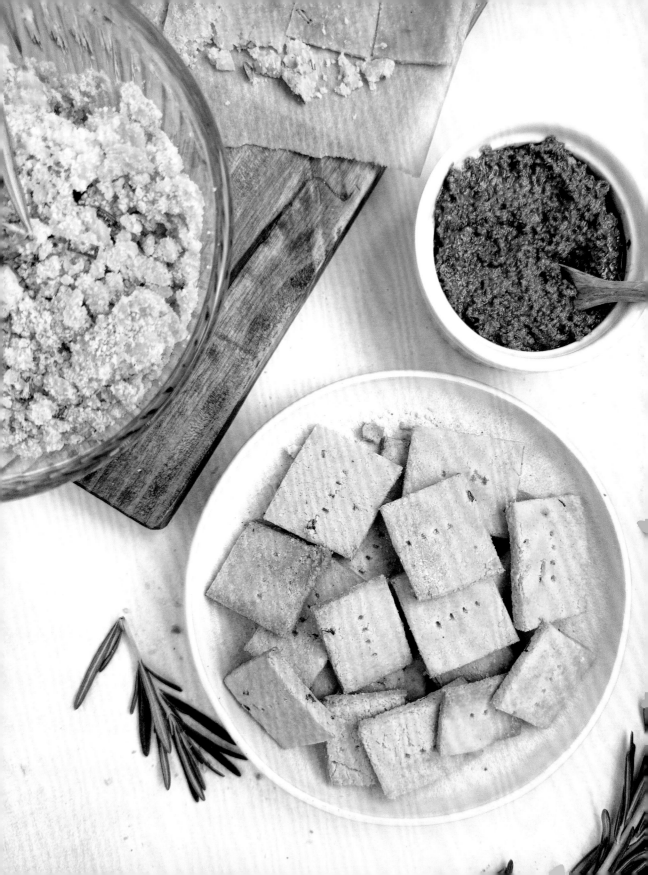

Roll the dough into a ball and then press the ball between two sheets of parchment paper to ⅛-inch thickness. You can use your hands or a rolling pin. Remove the top piece of parchment paper and transfer the bottom piece with the rolled-out dough to a baking sheet. Leaving it on the parchment paper, cut the dough into 2-inch squares with a knife or pizza cutter.

Bake until lightly golden, 12 to 15 minutes.

Sprinkle salt on top of crackers. Let the crackers cool on the baking sheet for 30 minutes before serving.

# SEVEN-LAYER DIP

*T*his dip is an all-time favorite for me, especially when paired with organic tortilla chips or Siete Dip Chips. Make it for yourself or take it to a party. Either way, I guarantee you won't be disappointed. When I make it for myself, I hold off on the olives and replace them with chopped avocado because olives aren't my thing. When I take the dip to a party, I make it as is, and it's always a big hit. The cashew queso dip can be swapped out for sour cream (like Good Culture). Feel free to make this dip your own in a way that your family and friends will most enjoy.

**SERVES 4**

. . . . . . . . . . . . . . . . . . . . . . . . . . . .

VEGETARIAN

One 15-ounce can organic pinto or black beans, rinsed and drained

1 large avocado

Juice of ½ lime

½ teaspoon sea salt

½ cup Cashew Queso Dip (page 159)

½ cup chopped romaine lettuce

¼ cup pickled jalapeños

½ cup diced seeded Roma tomatoes

¼ cup sliced black olives

2 tablespoons sliced green onion

FOR SERVING

Siete grain-free Dip Chips

Colorful, nonstarchy raw veggies, such as carrots, celery, cucumbers, radishes, snap peas, cherry tomatoes, broccoli, jicama, green beans, mushrooms, peppers, asparagus, and/or cauliflower

In a medium bowl, mash the beans with a fork and then spread the mashed beans evenly over the bottom of an 8 by 5-inch dish. Keep in mind, the bigger the dish, the thinner the layer will be.

In another medium bowl, mash the avocado with the lime juice and salt. Layer the smashed avocado on top of the beans, smoothing it out with a spatula.

Add the remaining layers in the following order: cashew queso dip, lettuce, jalapeños, tomatoes, black olives, and green onion.

Cover and refrigerate until ready to serve. Serve with tortilla chips and unlimited veggies.

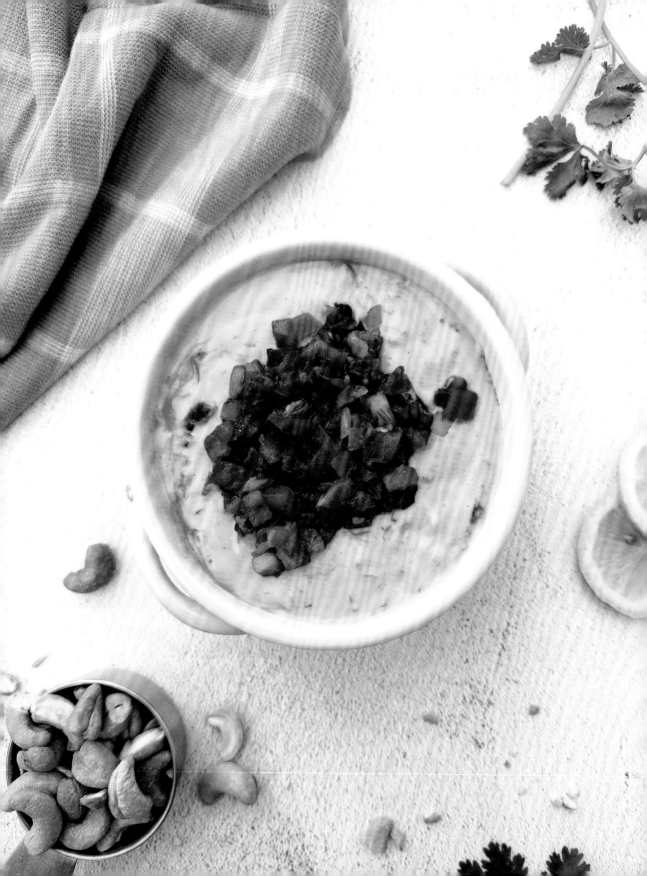

# CASHEW QUESO DIP

As I mentioned, you use this dip or sour cream in the Seven-Layer Dip. But I do hope you take the chance to make this queso dip to enjoy it on its own. It's so darn yummy as a dip or as a sauce. I've noticed a trend in some of my favorite recipes: They *must* qualify as both a sauce and a dip! This dip freezes pretty well, too, if you don't finish it all in one sitting.

### MAKES ABOUT 1½ CUPS

1 cup raw cashews, soaked for up to 4 hours and drained

1 teaspoon sea salt

¼ cup water

1½ tablespoons fresh lemon juice

3 tablespoons nutritional yeast

½ teaspoon ground turmeric

¼ to ½ cup salsa (mix in more for extra heat)

In a blender, combine the cashews, salt, water, lemon juice, yeast, turmeric, and salsa. Blend, adding more water if needed to get to your desired consistency.

# STUFFED SWEET POTATO

*T*his is such a great snack or meal to prep ahead of time. I honestly like sweet potatoes better leftover than I do fresh. I think it's because the flavor evolves after being cooked, similar to cake or soup. It's always better the next day, so bake a bunch ahead of time the next chance you get. This is a *sweet* stuffed sweet potato option, but you can always do savory, too. One of my favorite savory ways to eat a sweet potato is to stuff it with leftover chili. It's almost as to die for as this recipe.

**SERVES 1**
........................
VEGETARIAN

1 sweet potato, scrubbed

Sprinkle of pumpkin pie spice

Dash of sea salt

½ banana, sliced

1½ teaspoons flaxseed meal

1½ teaspoons hemp seeds

1½ teaspoons chia seeds

1 tablespoon chopped toasted hazelnuts, walnuts, or pecans

1 tablespoon pepitas

¼ cup gluten-free low-sugar granola (such as KIND) or homemade Granola (page 174)

1 tablespoon natural almond butter

½ teaspoon raw honey or pure maple syrup (optional)

Preheat the oven to 425°F.

Poke the sweet potato with a fork several times, then wrap the potato first with parchment paper and then with foil. Bake until soft, 45 to 50 minutes. You can cook the potato ahead of time.

Halve the cooked sweet potato and top with the pumpkin pie spice, salt, banana, flaxseed meal, hemp seeds, chia seeds, hazelnuts, pepitas, and granola. Drizzle almond butter over everything, then drizzle with honey (if using).

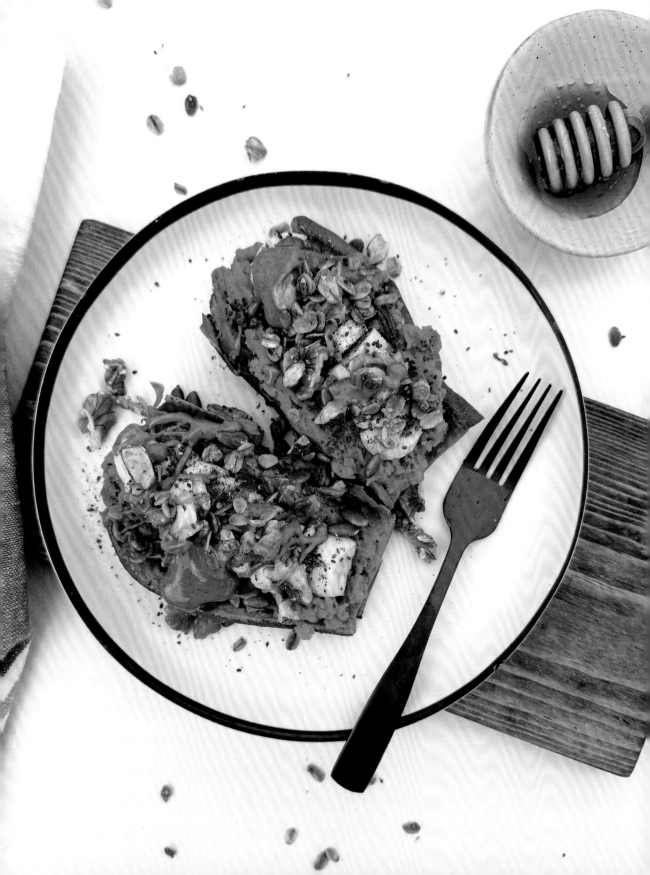

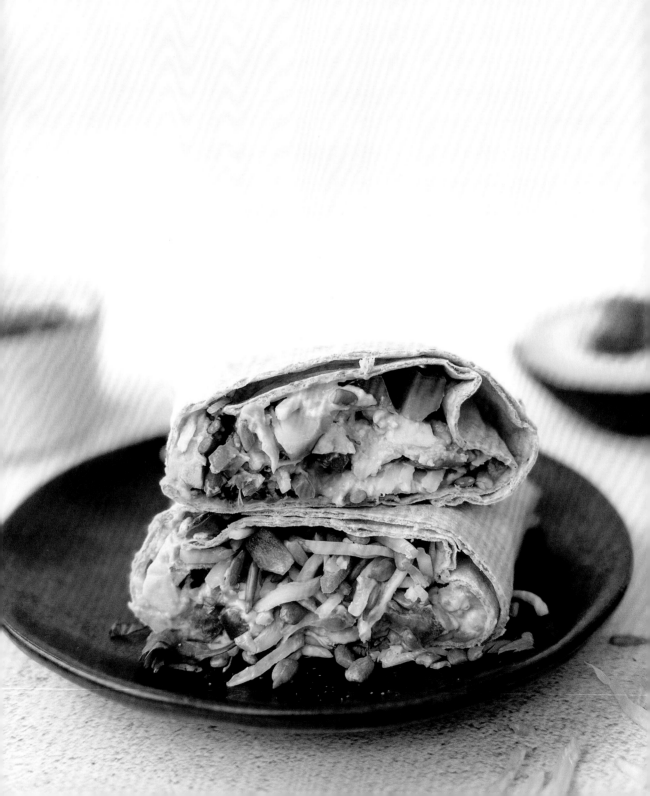

# VEGGIE HUMMUS WRAP

*D*o you have two minutes? That's all you need to put this combo together. The vegetables I use here are my favorites, but you can use any veggies you have on hand, and you could also swap the sunflower seeds for nuts or pepitas. This wrap is so delicious and filling, but as always, you get to be the judge of what's filling for you. If you're still hungry, have another one— that's what intuitive eating is!

**SERVES 1**
. . . . . . . . . . . . . . . . . . . . . . .

VEGETARIAN

2 tablespoons hummus

1 coconut wrap or Siete tortilla

1 tablespoon sunflower seeds

⅓ cup broccoli slaw mix

⅓ cup sliced red bell pepper

½ avocado, sliced

Spread the hummus on the wrap. Add the sunflower seeds, broccoli slaw, bell pepper, and avocado. Wrap to serve.

# CUCUMBER SALAD

*I*t's July as I'm writing this, and cucumbers are at the peak of their season where I live. My mouth is watering and I'm going to have to take a break to go make myself this recipe! There is something about the perfect amount of salt in the dressing that makes the cucumbers melt in your mouth. As long as you're using sea salt, you can add it according to your personal taste preference.

SERVES 4 TO 6
. . . . . . . . . . . . . . . . . . . . . . .
VEGETARIAN

2 English cucumbers, diced

1 pint cherry tomatoes, quartered

1 red onion, diced

1 tablespoon nutritional yeast

1 tablespoon sunflower seeds

DRESSING

2 tablespoons extra-virgin olive oil

1 tablespoon fresh lemon juice

1 tablespoon apple cider vinegar

½ teaspoon sea salt

½ teaspoon freshly ground black pepper

2 tablespoons minced fresh dill

In a large bowl, combine the cucumbers, tomatoes, onion, yeast, and sunflower seeds.

To make the dressing: In a small bowl, combine the olive oil, lemon juice, vinegar, salt, pepper, and dill. Whisk to combine.

Add the dressing to the salad and toss.

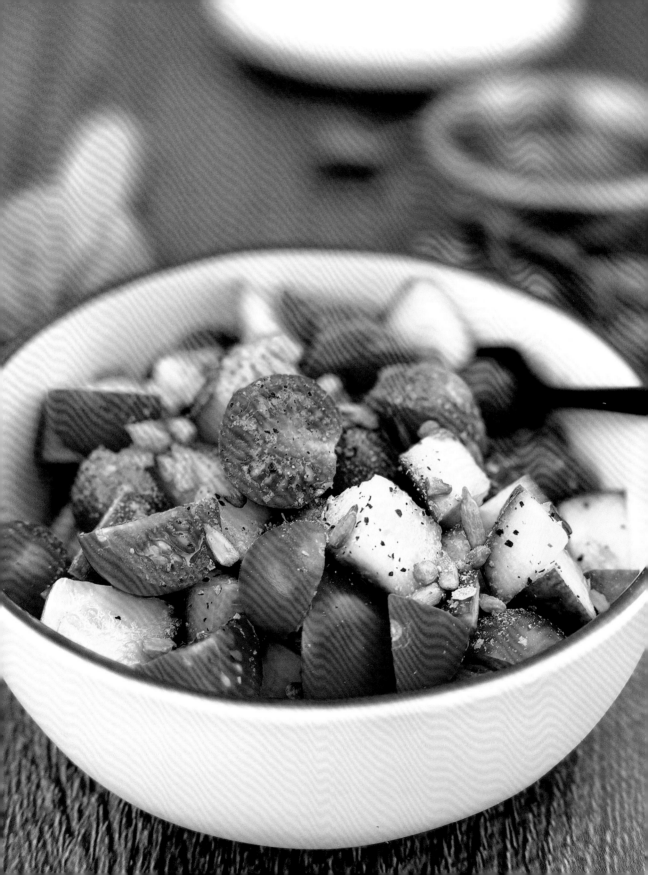

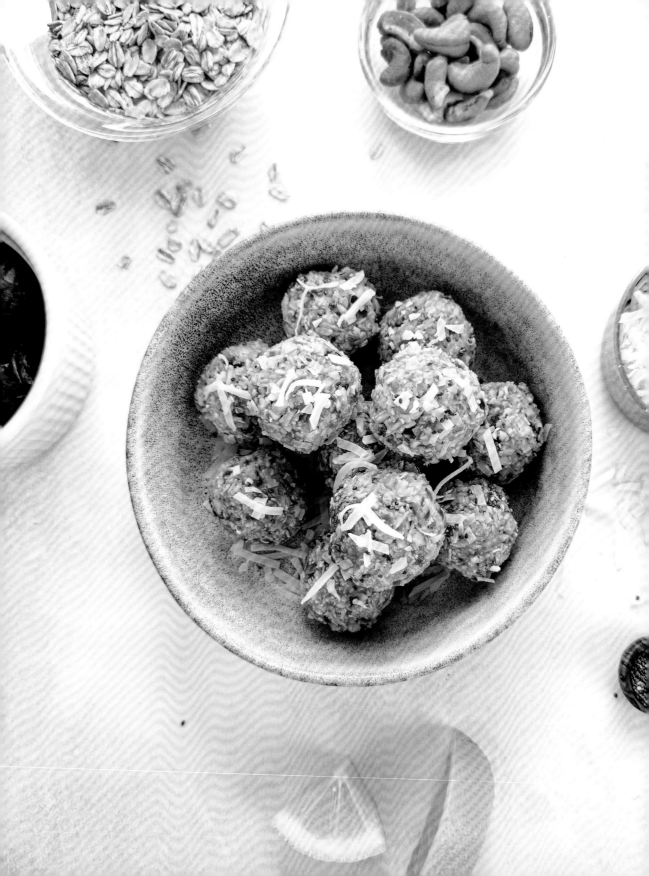

# CITRUS COCONUT BITES

*Y*ou'll be whisked away to the tropics with this snack. These energy bites are simple to make, with a great flavor, but the nutrients in them are anything but simple. Coconut is another one of my personal superfoods, boasting loads of trace minerals as well as medium-chain tri-glycerides (MCTs). MCTs are fats that are metabolized more quickly than other fatty acids, so you can use them for energy with less chance of any of the fat being stored in your body. As you pulse the dough for these bites in the food processor, be sure the oils are seeping out from the cashews and coconut so the dough is easy to roll.

**MAKES ABOUT 16 BITES**

**VEGETARIAN**

1¼ cups unsweetened shredded coconut

½ cup cashews

½ cup rolled oats or gluten-free oats

½ cup pitted dates

Grated zest of 1 lemon

Juice of 1 to 2 lemons (depending on how much lemon flavor you'd like)

½ teaspoon poppy seeds

In a food processor, combine 1 cup of the coconut, the cashews, oats, dates, lemon zest, lemon juice, and poppy seeds. Pulse until well combined and somewhat sticky. Form the dough into balls and roll in the remaining ¼ cup coconut. Store in an airtight container in the refrigerator for up to 1 week.

# EASY FERMENTED VEGGIES

*Y*ou may consider saying goodbye to store-bought pickles after this recipe hits your home. You know how you can pretty much fry anything? The same goes for pickling, and this fermented veggie recipe takes advantage of that fact. If you're a gardener, this is a tasty way to preserve your veggies at the end of a season. Store them up to 4 months in the refrigerator. Even if you don't garden, this is a great method for cutting down on food waste. Stock up on your seasonings below and never throw out a veggie again.

**SERVES 3 OR 4**

VEGETARIAN

Several sprigs dill

1 teaspoon celery seeds

1 teaspoon coriander seeds

1 teaspoon mustard seeds

1 teaspoon peppercorns (black or tricolor)

2 jalapeño chiles, quartered (for less spice, remove membrane and seeds)

4 cups water

8 garlic cloves, peeled but whole

2 cups distilled white vinegar

6 teaspoons Himalayan pink salt

6 pickling cucumbers, quartered lengthwise

4 rainbow carrots, peeled and cut into thick matchsticks, similar in length to the cucumbers

Handful of green beans, ends trimmed

3 radishes, sliced

Set out four 1-pint or two 1-quart mason jars with the lids. Divide the dill sprigs, celery seeds, coriander seeds, mustard seeds, peppercorns, and jalapeño pieces among the jars.

In a medium saucepan, bring the water to a boil. Reduce to a simmer, add the garlic, and cook for 5 minutes. Add the vinegar and salt and increase the heat to bring the mixture to a boil, stirring until the salt dissolves. Remove from the heat.

With a slotted spoon, remove the garlic. Divide the garlic among the jars. Pack the jars with the cucumbers, carrots, green beans, and radishes, stacking the veggies vertically and stuffing them in as tightly as you can.

Bring the brine back to a boil, then carefully pour it over the vegetables in the jars to cover them completely, leaving about a ½-inch space from the top of each jar. Seal the jars, let them cool, and refrigerate.

The pickles will be ready to eat by the next day, and the flavor will get even better over the next few days. Each jar keeps about 3 months in the fridge.

**NOTE:** To make Spicy Pickled Green Beans, follow the steps above, using all green beans (or a mix of green and yellow) instead of the mixed veggies, double the jalapeños, and add ½ teaspoon red pepper flakes to the bottom of each jar.

# DARK CHOCOLATE ZUCCHINI BLENDER MUFFINS

*T*hese have been a longtime hit in our family. For one thing, my dad always grows enough zucchini for an entire village. We end up with hefty amounts, and like other squash, this vegetable has a short shelf life. I'm not trying to sneak a vegetable into a treat here—the vegetable actually makes the recipe so moist that it will melt in your mouth. These muffins just wouldn't be the same without the zucchini.

**MAKES 10 MUFFINS**

½ cup canned pumpkin puree

½ cup natural almond butter

1 egg

1 teaspoon pure vanilla extract

¼ cup cacao powder

¼ cup raw honey

1 teaspoon baking soda

Dash of sea salt

½ large zucchini, shredded and squeezed dry with a clean kitchen towel (about 1 cup)

⅓ cup mini dark chocolate chips

Preheat the oven to 375°F. Line 10 cups of a muffin tin with paper liners or use silicone muffin cups.

In a blender, combine the pumpkin puree, almond butter, egg, vanilla, cacao powder, honey, baking soda, and salt and blend. Fold in the zucchini. Pour the batter into the muffin cups, filling them three-quarters full. Top with the chocolate chips.

Bake until a toothpick comes out clean, 20 to 25 minutes.

Let the muffins cool at least 10 minutes before removing them from the pan.

# VEGGIE QUINOA BITES

Serve on a tray for your kids . . . or save them all for yourself. If you eat dairy, you will love this recipe as is. If you don't do dairy, the yeast swap will make all your nondairy dreams come true! These are so good either way. Did you know that quinoa falls into the "complete protein" category? That means it contains all nine essential amino acids that our bodies don't make. Wild, right? It's one of the very few plant-based foods in that category. Amino acids are required for the synthesis of body protein and some neurotransmitters. Our bodies naturally create amino acids, but there are nine we need to get from our diet, which is why they are called *essential*. I have a feeling this recipe will become an essential part of your snacking rotation!

**SERVES 8**

Oil, for the muffin tin

1 cup uncooked quinoa

1 egg

1 cup diced onion

½ cup finely chopped broccoli

½ cup finely chopped cauliflower

3 garlic cloves, finely chopped or minced

1 cup spinach

½ cup organic shredded cheddar cheese or nutritional yeast

½ teaspoon dried parsley

½ teaspoon sea salt

½ teaspoon freshly ground black pepper

Chopped green onion, for garnish

Preheat the oven to 350°F. Lightly grease 8 cups of a muffin tin with oil.

Cook the quinoa according to the package directions. Drain well.

In a large bowl or in the pot the quinoa was cooked in, combine the quinoa, egg, onion, broccoli, cauliflower, garlic, spinach, cheddar, parsley, salt, and pepper.

Scoop about ¼ cup of the mixture into each muffin cup and slightly flatten it.

Bake until lightly browned on top, about 20 minutes. Allow to cool slightly before serving. Garnish with chopped green onion.

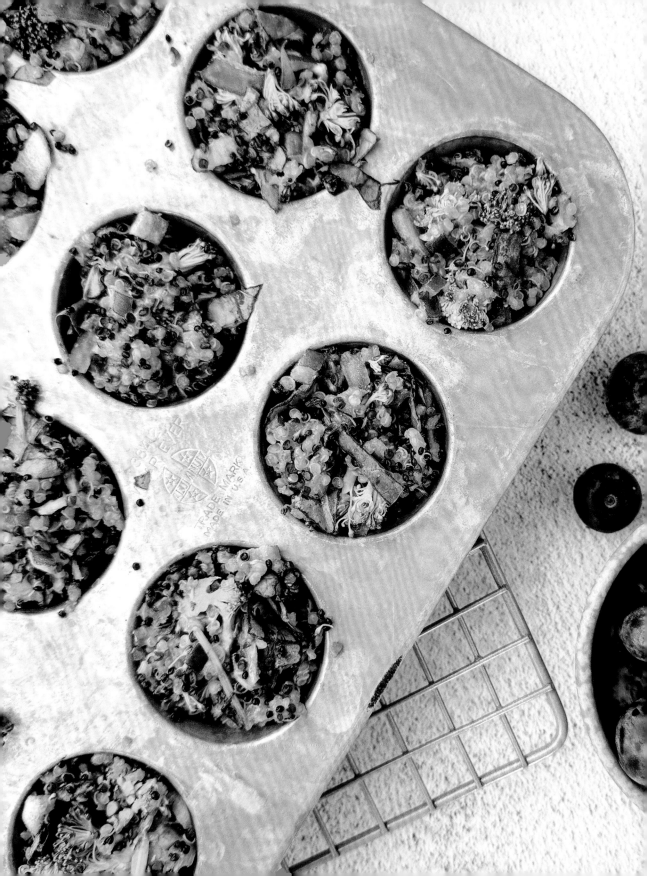

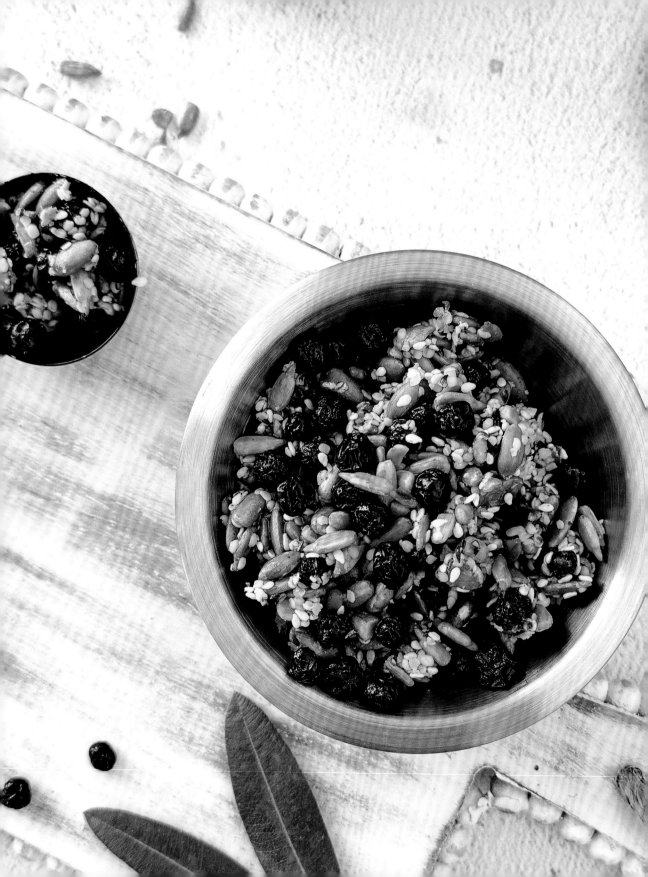

# SUPER SEED TRAIL MIX

*P*eople always ask me what snacks I keep on hand in case I get caught without food for longer than the 4-hour window. Trail mix or mixed nuts has always been that food for me, especially when I'm traveling. Seeds generally pass the test for allergies, so it's a safer bet to travel with the super seed trail mix rather than nuts. At home, I store this mix in a jar, and when I'm on the go, I take it with me in a silicone bag. It's super easy to make with the slightest hint of sweetness, and the dried fruit can be just the carb fill you need to sustain your energy levels.

**SERVES 4**

VEGETARIAN

½ cup sunflower seeds

½ cup pepitas

¼ cup sesame seeds

¼ cup hemp seeds

¼ cup dried chopped cherries or other unsweetened dried berry

1 teaspoon raw honey, warmed

In a large bowl, combine the sunflower seeds, pepitas, sesame seeds, hemp seeds, and cherries. Add the honey and mix to combine, letting the honey bind the small seeds to the larger ones.

**NOTE:** If you'd like to roast the trail mix, preheat the oven to 325°F and line a baking sheet with parchment paper. Spread the mix on the pan and bake for 12 minutes. Roasting is not necessary, but it does create a crispier trail mix that lasts longer.

# GRANOLA

*T*his might be another recipe that causes you to stop buying the store-bought version. I store ours in a jar, and my girls enjoy it by the handful, on their yogurt, and as a topping for their smoothie bowls. But it came about as a complete accident. We needed granola to top an acai bowl and we were out, so I had to think fast and create something I knew my girls would love. It worked!

**SERVES 4**

VEGETARIAN

2 cups rolled oats or gluten-free oats

½ cup sliced almonds

1 tablespoon chia seeds

3 tablespoons coconut oil, melted

⅓ cup pure maple syrup

1 tablespoon pumpkin pie spice

¼ cup natural almond butter

1 teaspoon pure vanilla extract

½ teaspoon sea salt

Preheat the oven to 325°F. Line a baking sheet with parchment paper or a silicone mat.

In a large bowl, combine the oats, almonds, chia seeds, coconut oil, maple syrup, pumpkin pie spice, almond butter, vanilla, and salt. Stir to combine. Pour the granola onto the prepared baking sheet and pat it down to create one even layer.

Bake for 20 minutes. Rotate the pan front to back and bake until the granola is golden and fragrant, another 3 to 5 minutes.

Let it cool completely before serving or storing. Granola can be stored in an airtight container in a cool, dry spot for up to 1 month. You can also freeze it for up to 6 months in a resealable freezer bag.

**NOTE:** For a delicious snack, serve granola over ½ cup berries and ¼ cup unsweetened nondairy milk.

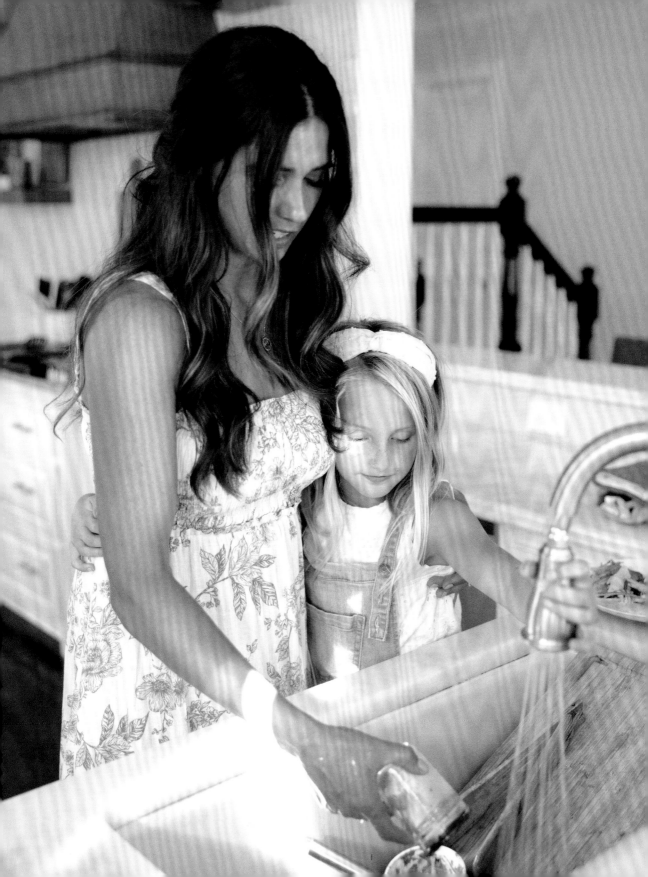

# YOGURT PARFAIT

*I*'ve included this parfait in the snack chapter, but at our house, it's a highly requested breakfast dish as well. The seasoned and sautéed apple is so delicious, taking on a deeper flavor that some foods get with slight cooking. If you're dairy-free, there are thankfully a plethora of yogurt varieties you can use. I prefer a coconut-based version, but there are almond- and cashew-based yogurts as well. Just be sure to add some protein if you're going the dairy-free route. I like to use collagen peptides in that scenario.

**SERVES 1**

VEGETARIAN

1 small apple, diced

1 teaspoon ghee or coconut oil

⅔ cup 2% or whole-milk Greek yogurt

4 tablespoons low-sugar clean granola (such as Purely Elizabeth) or homemade Granola (page 174)

Sprinkle of ground cinnamon, about ¼ teaspoon

1 tablespoon chopped pecans or walnuts

In a small skillet, sauté the apple in the ghee until soft, about 8 minutes. Set aside to cool.

Place the yogurt in a glass, jar, or bowl. On top of the yogurt, layer the apples, granola, cinnamon, and pecans.

**NOTE:** Another option is to add fresh berries on top of the yogurt, instead of the apples.

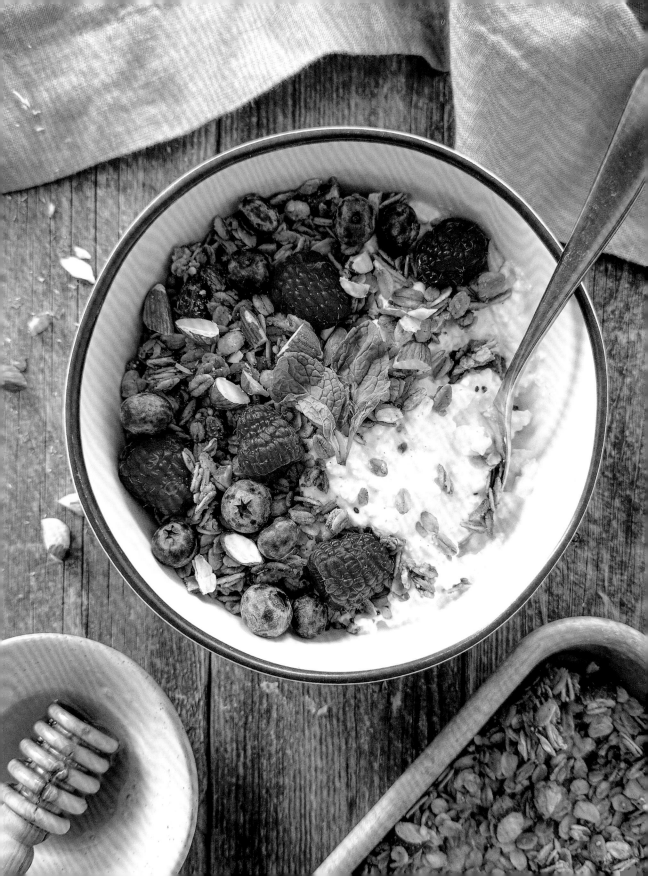

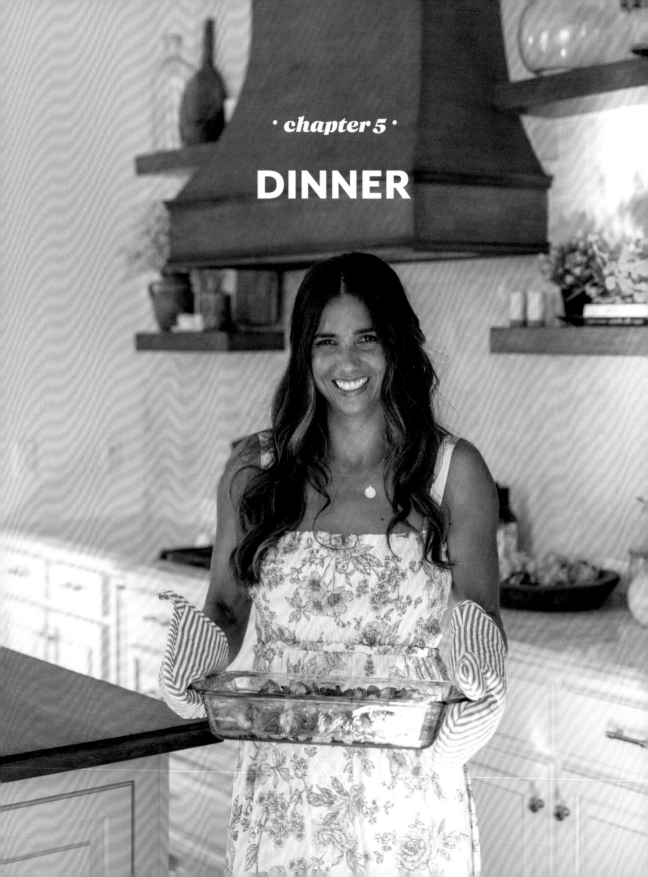

· chapter 5 ·

# DINNER

**As you prepare** dinner for your family, I invite you to sit in the presence of what the day has brought. By "sit in," I mean being mindful as you prepare dinner. Take note of the shift in your nutrition. Has it enabled you to manage stress differently? Maybe now that your body and mind are better nourished, you're slower to anger. Maybe you've noticed yourself in a better mood. Maybe you are experiencing better mental clarity. Maybe tasks like dinner prep don't seem as daunting. Be present and reflect on these changes. The kitchen is a place to feel nurtured and nourished, even if you're the one putting in most of the work. It's not for nothing!

At the table, ask your family what their highs and lows of the day were. Share yours as well. Parents, we are all human—it's okay to share our struggles along with our wins. I used to be wary of sharing my struggles with my kids, but as they got older, I realized if I want them to share with *me,* I need to be transparent with *them*. And honestly, the kitchen is where so much of this conversation, heartache, joy, and victory is shared.

I like to think of dinner as a form of church. We are gathering together daily and reconnecting as a family the same way we, as part of our church family, gather and reconnect on Sundays. Matthew 18:20 reads, "For where two or three are gathered together in my name, there am I in the midst of them." At the dinner table together, my husband, kids, and I bless the meal and the people who will share it. We recite our family dinner prayer together, and on Sundays we usually call on one of our kids to offer some extra words of prayer. There are few greater blessings than sharing meals together as a family, and I encourage you to do this as much as possible.

Of course, dinner is also an opportunity to provide your family with a nourishing last meal of the day, to improve their health and prepare their bodies for a good night's sleep that will restore them on a cellular level. In my opinion, a good healthy dinner sets the stage for a good, restful sleep. Our bodies are always working, even when we aren't. A healthy dinner fuels that work!

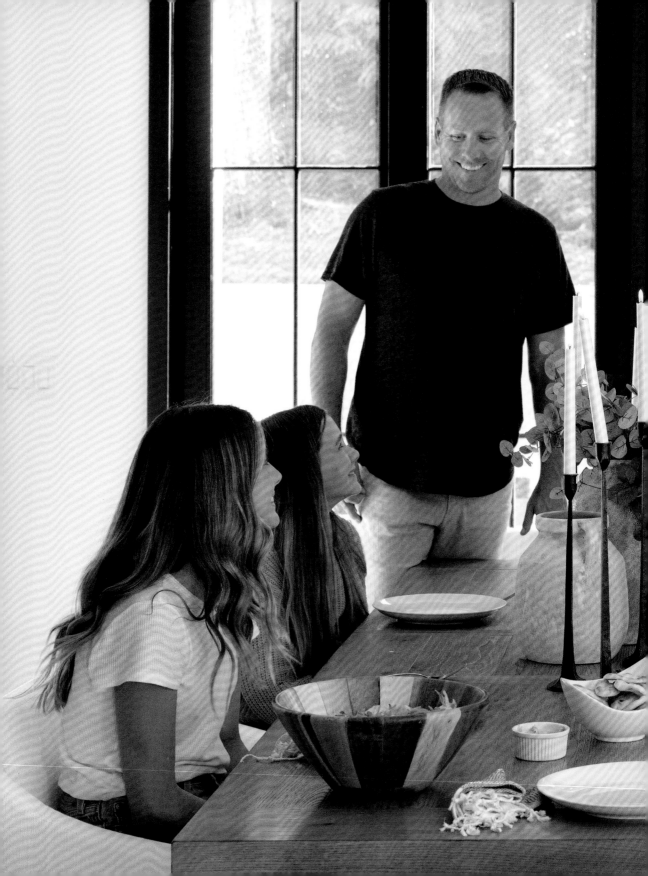

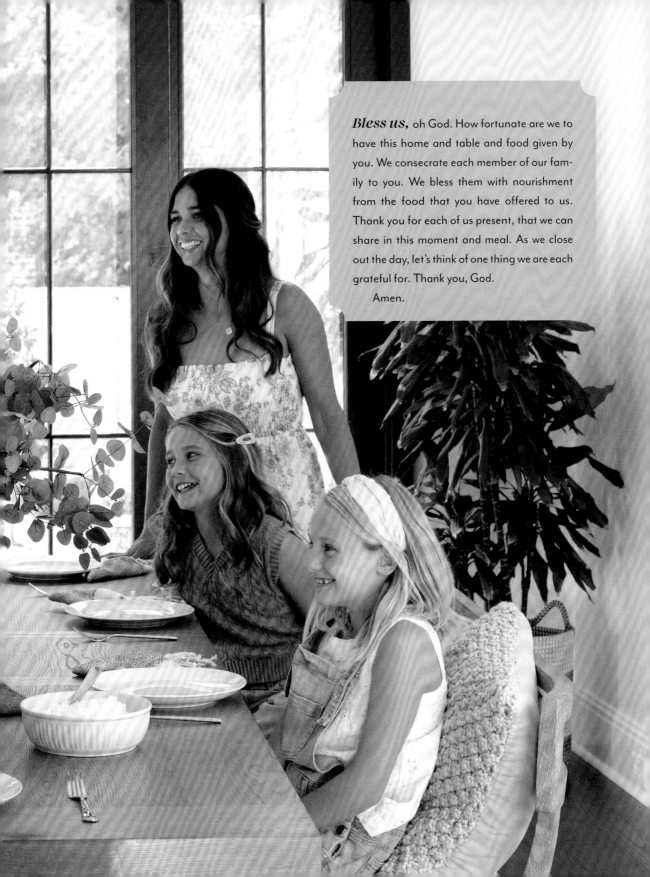

**Bless us,** oh God. How fortunate are we to have this home and table and food given by you. We consecrate each member of our family to you. We bless them with nourishment from the food that you have offered to us. Thank you for each of us present, that we can share in this moment and meal. As we close out the day, let's think of one thing we are each grateful for. Thank you, God.

Amen.

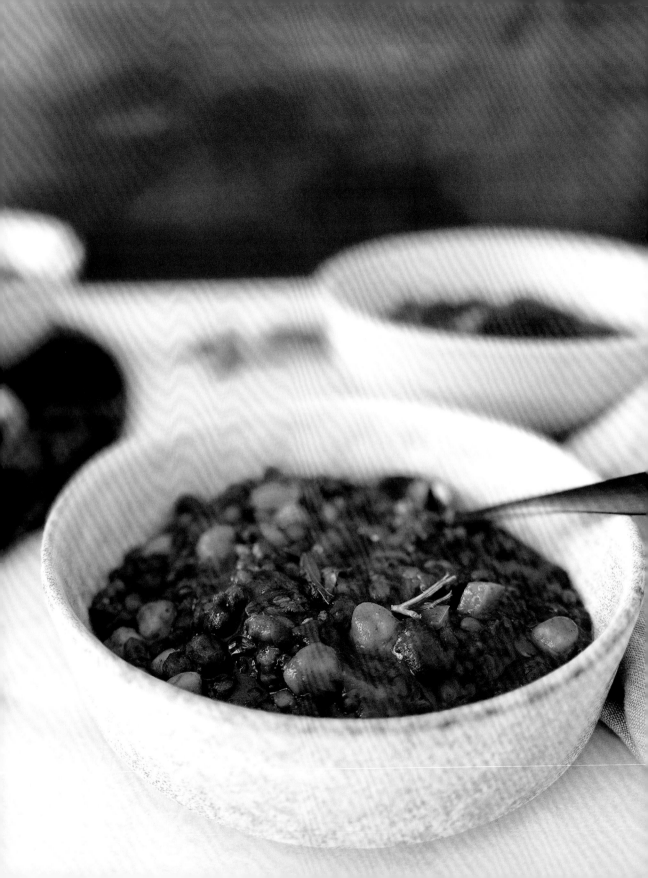

# SUPERFOOD CHILI

**SERVES 8**

VEGETARIAN, BUT YOU CAN
ADD GROUND TURKEY OR
CHICKEN IF YOU'D LIKE.

1 cup chopped onion

1 cup chopped carrots

1 cup chopped celery

1 cup chopped green bell
pepper

4 garlic cloves, minced

One 15-ounce can organic
lentils, undrained

One 15-ounce can organic
chickpeas, undrained

One 15-ounce can
organic kidney beans,
undrained

One 15-ounce can organic
pinto beans, undrained

One 6-ounce can organic
tomato paste

6 Roma tomatoes, cut into
chunks

2 teaspoons chili powder

2 teaspoons ground cumin

1 pound lean ground
organic turkey
or chicken breast
(optional; for added
protein)

Himalayan pink salt and
freshly ground black
pepper

Vegetable or bone broth (if
needed for more liquid)

*T*his veggie-loaded chili can become your go-to when you're craving a chili dinner. With all the fiber-packed, nutrient-dense foods in this recipe, don't be surprised if your eyes are bigger than your tummy. That's okay! Remember, intuitive eating helps us evaluate by the meal what we need for energy. While we have suggested servings listed with each recipe, your serving size is dependent on you. You get to decide how much you can and want to eat. There are two versions here: one for the stovetop and one for a slow cooker.

**STOVETOP CHILI**

In a large soup pot or Dutch oven, combine the onion, carrots, celery, bell pepper, garlic, lentils, chickpeas, kidney beans, pinto beans, tomato paste, tomatoes, chili powder, cumin, ground turkey (if using), and salt and black pepper to taste. Cover and simmer over medium-low heat for 1 hour, stirring occasionally. If more liquid is needed, add broth.

**SLOW COOKER CHILI**

In a slow cooker, combine the onion, carrots, celery, bell pepper, garlic, lentils, chickpeas, kidney beans, pinto beans, tomato paste, tomatoes, chili powder, cumin, ground turkey (if using), and salt and black pepper to taste. Cook on low for 4 to 6 hours.

**NOTE:** You can use dried beans instead of canned. Soak them overnight before using.

# CREAMY LEMON CHICKEN SOUP

SERVES 4 OR 5

TO MAKE VEGETARIAN, OMIT THE CHICKEN AND SUBSTITUTE TWO 15-OUNCE CANS ORGANIC CANNELLINI BEANS, RINSED AND DRAINED. USE VEGETABLE BROTH INSTEAD OF BONE BROTH.

1 tablespoon avocado oil (for the Instant Pot version)

2 carrots, peeled and sliced

1 small yellow or white onion, chopped

4 celery stalks, chopped

1 cup chopped zucchini or yellow squash

1 pound mini potatoes, quartered

4 garlic cloves, minced

1 teaspoon dried oregano

1 teaspoon Italian seasoning

½ teaspoon ground turmeric

1 tablespoon sea salt

1 teaspoon freshly ground black pepper

1 bay leaf

1½ pounds boneless, skinless chicken breasts (or half breasts and half thighs)

4 cups chicken bone broth or vegetable broth

⅓ cup fresh lemon juice

⅓ cup Kite Hill almond milk cream cheese

Something that has never made much sense to me is soup being deemed only a winter or colder-month food. I get that our bodies crave warming foods during these months, but my body craves soup even on a warm summer day. And here's the thing, most evenings, no matter what time of year it is, the dinner you eat is going to be warm, unless it's a salad or the meal has already gotten cold. So why can't soup be considered year-round? Don't be afraid to make this easy lemon chicken soup any day of the year. The bright lemony flavor with the summer zucchini or yellow squash is like a warm taste of sunshine. There are two versions here: one for a slow cooker and one for an Instant Pot.

**SLOW COOKER CREAMY LEMON SOUP**

In a slow cooker, combine the carrots, onion, celery, zucchini, potatoes, garlic, oregano, Italian seasoning, turmeric, salt, pepper, bay leaf, chicken, and broth. Cover and cook on high for 3 hours or low for 5 to 6 hours.

Remove the chicken and shred it with two forks. (Alternatively, use a stand or hand mixer to shred the chicken). Return the shredded chicken to the slow cooker and add the lemon juice and cream cheese. Stir until the cream cheese is melted into the soup and everything is well combined. Taste and adjust seasonings if needed. Discard the bay leaf.

Serve garnished with black pepper and parsley, with lemon wedges for squeezing.

**INSTANT POT CREAMY LEMON SOUP**

Select the Sauté function. Drizzle the oil in the bottom of the pot. Add the carrots, onion, celery, zucchini, and potatoes. Sauté for 3 minutes. Add the garlic, oregano, Italian season-

Freshly ground black
  pepper

Chopped fresh parsley

Lemon wedges, for
  squeezing

ing, turmeric, salt, and pepper. Sauté for another minute. Add the bay leaf, chicken, and broth. Cancel the Sauté.

Cover, seal, and cook on high pressure for 10 minutes. Let the pressure release naturally.

Carefully remove the lid, remove the chicken, and shred with two forks. (Alternatively, use a stand or hand mixer to shred the chicken.) Return the shredded chicken to the Instant Pot and add the lemon juice and cream cheese. Stir until the cream cheese is melted into the soup and everything is well combined. Taste and adjust seasonings if needed. Discard the bay leaf.

Serve garnished with the black pepper and parsley, with lemon wedges for squeezing.

# CABBAGE SOUP

SERVES 4
..........................
VEGETARIAN

2 tablespoons avocado oil

1 cup chopped yellow
onion

2 garlic cloves, diced or
pressed

1 cup sliced mushrooms

1 teaspoon Himalayan pink
salt

1 teaspoon freshly ground
black pepper

4 cups tomato sauce

8 cups vegetable broth or
bone broth

Two 15-ounce cans organic
chickpeas or cannellini
beans, rinsed and
drained

1 teaspoon Trader Joe's
21 Seasoning Salute or
Italian seasoning

2 teaspoons ground
turmeric

2 small zucchini, quartered
lengthwise and cut
crosswise into ¼-inch
pieces

3 cups shredded cabbage
(can use red and green
cabbage for more color
benefits)

2 large carrots, peeled and
sliced into ¼-inch pieces

1 cup green beans, ends
trimmed

Cabbage soup has gotten a bad rap over the years for being part of diets or liquid-based cleanses. Back when I was getting into the nutrition world, the culture was very pro calorie restriction. Like all cruciferous vegetables, cabbage is high fiber and super filling while boasting low calories, making it a popular ingredient in diet recipes at the time. I challenged myself to create a nutrient-dense, filling version of cabbage soup that doesn't make you feel like you're on a diet. With a plethora of other foods added and a jazzed-up tomato-sauce base, this soup is delicious, satisfying, and filled to the brim with ready-to-use nutrients. I love this one as leftovers as much as I love it fresh.

Heat a large Dutch oven or large soup pot over medium heat and add the oil. Add the onion and garlic and sauté for 3 minutes. Stir in the mushrooms and sprinkle with the salt and pepper.

Add the tomato sauce, broth, chickpeas, 21 Seasoning Salute, turmeric, zucchini, cabbage, carrots, and green beans and bring to a quick boil. Reduce to a simmer and cook, stirring occasionally, until the vegetables are soft, about 40 minutes.

## FEEL-GOOD FAQ

### What about alcohol?

The dreaded question! I'm not against the occasional drink. That being said, don't forget our guiding principle: feeling good!

Alcohol is not a food—it's not as simple as calories in and calories out. Protein and carbs carry 4 calories per gram. Fat carries 9 calories per gram, which is why we say it's twice as energy dense. Alcohol has its own profile, carrying 7 calories per gram. It's not energizing like fat is, and it doesn't work for us on a cellular level, so that's 7 calories per gram that we have to get out of our bodies before we can burn energy effectively again. Even if you aren't choosing sugary mixers, you are still ingesting calories that aren't nourishing. Not only that, alcohol inhibits natural detoxification while it's in our system. It's also dehydrating, leading to that not-so-good feeling at night and the next morning.

I try to stay disciplined around my own drinking, choosing when and how much I want to indulge based on how it's going to make me feel. As a basic rule of thumb, I stick to no more than one to three glasses of anything a week. If you're trying to heal, alcohol should really be cut out or saved for only special occasions. You are the judge of how you feel, so let that be your guide, and always drink lots of water no matter what else you are drinking!

Once you begin to feel good after implementing the Feel-Good philosophy in your everyday life, you may notice more side effects than you used to from what you drink. You may notice skin irritation, digestive issues, brain fog, or overall lack of mental clarity. You may notice achy joints or random pain. These side effects lead to us making even better choices!

# LOADED RED SKIN POTATOES

SERVES 4

TO MAKE VEGETARIAN, OMIT THE TURKEY AND USE 2 CUPS STEAMED LENTILS (I LOVE TRADER JOE'S) INSTEAD.

3 tablespoons avocado oil

One 1-ounce packet clean taco seasoning (such as Siete), or 2 tablespoons Homemade Taco Seasoning (recipe follows)

2 tablespoons water

5 medium red or gold potatoes, cut into wedges

1 pound ground organic turkey

One 15-ounce can organic pinto beans, drained

One 15-ounce jar Siete Red Enchilada Sauce

1 teaspoon garlic powder

1 teaspoon chili powder

1 teaspoon onion powder

Sea salt and freshly ground black pepper

One 15-ounce jar Siete Cashew Queso or homemade Cashew Queso Dip (page 159)

Chopped green onions, for garnish

*P*otatoes are some of the most versatile foods around if you think outside the box. For so long, when carbs were getting a bad rap, people stopped eating potatoes. Maybe it's the Midwesterner in me, but I could never give up potatoes—I just find ways to make them healthier. Here's a fun fact: Red and yellow potatoes contain what's called "resistant starch." Resistant starches act like soluble fiber and resist part of the digestion process, helping with insulin levels, fat storage, and glucose. Long story short: Don't give up on foods that grow in the earth until you have the full picture!

Preheat the oven to 375°F.

In a large bowl, combine 2 tablespoons of the avocado oil, the taco seasoning, and water. Mix well. Add the potatoes and toss to mix. Spread the potatoes on a baking sheet.

Bake until tender, 30 to 40 minutes.

Meanwhile, in a large skillet, heat the remaining 1 tablespoon avocado oil over medium heat. Add the turkey and cook until browned, about 10 minutes. Add the beans and enchilada sauce and bring to a simmer. Add the garlic powder, chili powder, onion powder, and salt and pepper to taste. Simmer for 10 minutes to thicken the sauce slightly.

Heat the cashew queso according to the package directions.

To serve, scoop the chili sauce over the potato wedges, then top with queso. Garnish with the green onions.

3 tablespoons ground
  cumin

1 tablespoon garlic powder

1 tablespoon onion powder

1 tablespoon chili powder

¼ to 1 teaspoon cayenne
  pepper, to taste

1 teaspoon sea salt

¼ teaspoon freshly ground
  black pepper

## HOMEMADE TACO SEASONING

I have a jar of this seasoning sitting in my pantry at all times, and not just for tacos. I also add it to fajitas, chili, and any Tex-Mex meal I make. I've never found just the right flavor combo at stores, so I prefer to make my own and keep it on hand.

In a small bowl, stir together all the ingredients. Transfer to an airtight container to store for up to 2 months.

## FEEL-GOOD FAQ

**Should I give up on going out to restaurants, or is there a way to eat out and stay within the Feel-Good Way guidelines? I don't want to backslide!**

For a long time, I didn't eat out at restaurants because I always felt bad afterward—both physically, because of the food choices I made, and also emotionally, because I felt bad about myself for making those choices. All of which added up to no fun. But, when it comes to food, nothing is more important than feeling good. Once I focused on feeling good, I was able to start making the right choices even when eating out. I was able to imagine myself later that night trying to sleep and how my digestion might be, how I might feel waking up in the morning, depending on which food and drinks I chose. At some point, feeling good for the next several hours and the following day won out over momentary pleasure, and I was able to trust my choices.

You can enjoy yourself at a restaurant *and* still feel good that night and in the morning. I also set the mental tone of the 80/20 rule. If we stick with our very best food choices 80 percent of the time, then 20 percent of the time, we can indulge a little. For me personally, even if I'm veering into the 20 percent territory, I still try to choose veggie-loaded meals instead of meat-dominant dishes with few vegetables, and stay within food choices that I know will make me feel good. And if everyone is sharing dessert, I'll have a bite. But I don't ever order my own!

**MY FEEL-GOOD TIPS FOR EATING OUT**

- Choose a restaurant that can accommodate your Feel-Good needs. At some point, once you've become accustomed to feeling good, it's really not worth it to go backward, especially when you know what you're doing and what's going to happen. Restaurants that don't specialize in the kind of food you've grown accustomed to often have at least a few menu items that can fit, especially if you ask for slight modifications.

- Check the menu before you go, so you're informed about your options and not caught in indecision, which can lead to throwing in the towel and feeling bad later.

- If you order a salad, get the dressing on the side and use the amount that is best for you rather than the restaurant standard.

- Feel free to ask for extra vegetables, to hold the bread, or make other adjustments to meet your needs.

- Be sure you're hydrated before you even leave the house.

- Be thoughtful and sparing with alcohol.

There's nothing better than finding a restaurant where you can enjoy yourself *and* feel good! So do some restaurant shopping and find that Feel-Good spot you can return to when you need to take a break from your own kitchen.

# HEARTY CHICKEN POT PIE STEW

**SERVES 6**

TO MAKE VEGETARIAN, OMIT
THE CHICKEN, ADD 1 CUP
CHOPPED MUSHROOMS,
AND USE VEGETABLE BROTH
INSTEAD OF CHICKEN BROTH.

¼ cup avocado oil

1 yellow onion, chopped

2 celery stalks, chopped

½ cup chopped carrots

3 garlic cloves, or more to
taste, minced

3 red potatoes, diced

¼ cup non-GMO
cornstarch or arrowroot
flour

One 32-ounce box
organic chicken broth,
vegetable broth, or
bone broth

⅓ cup coconut milk

1½ teaspoons chopped
fresh thyme

2 cups shredded cooked
chicken (home-
poached in broth or
store-bought organic
rotisserie chicken)

½ cup frozen green beans

1 cup frozen peas

½ cup frozen corn kernels

Sea salt and freshly ground
black pepper

*I* can't remember the last time I ate pot pie. The heaviness just doesn't typically sit well with me. I have always loved the heartiness and flavors of it, though, so a few years ago, I set out to create the same taste and feeling of chicken pot pie but without the same "after-feelings." This stew is so satisfying in warm or cool months, and it always pleases a crowd. My kids and husband request it year-round, and it's a great, healthful meal to bring someone recovering from surgery or having a baby.

In a large soup pot, heat the oil over medium heat. Add the onion, celery, and carrots and cook until tender, about 10 minutes.

Add the garlic and potatoes, sprinkle with the cornstarch, and stir until the veggies are coated and the cornstarch starts to dissolve. Stir in the broth, coconut milk, and thyme. Reduce the heat to low and simmer until the potatoes are tender, about 20 minutes.

Stir in the chicken, green beans, peas, and corn and cook until heated through. Season with salt and pepper.

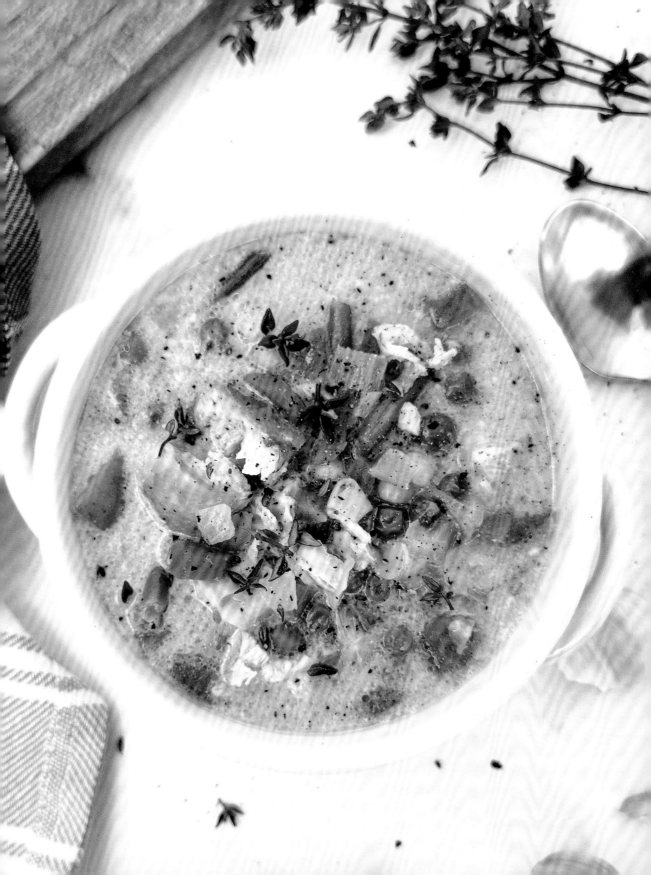

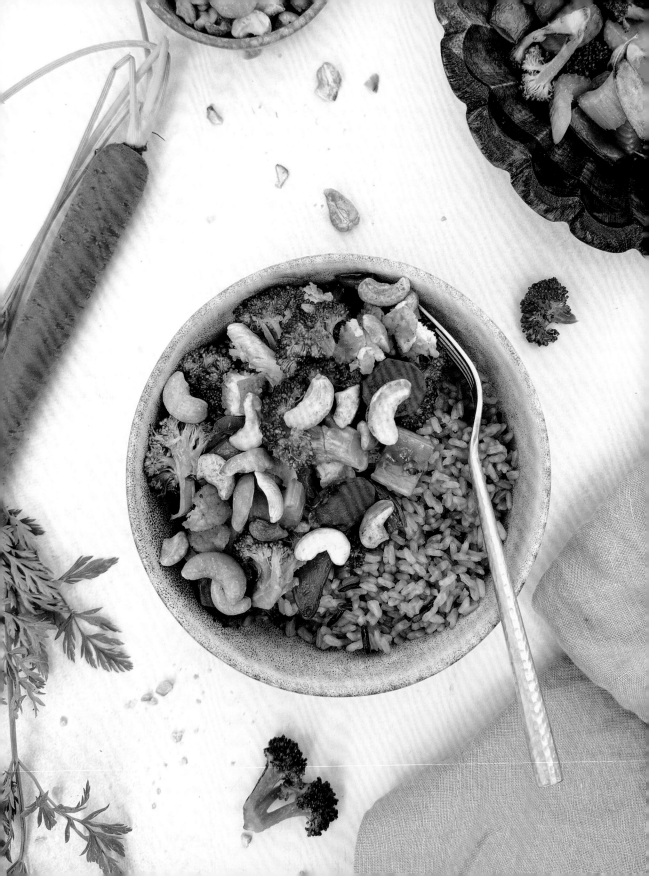

# SIMPLE STIR-FRY

With four active daughters, our after-school hours slip away quickly, so I lean in to fast weeknight meals like stir-fry. This simple one is a kid-pleaser at our house. When my kids request it, they almost always ask me to add chicken sausage. If your schedule is like ours, think about adding this recipe to your quick weeknight meal menu.

**SERVES 4**

........................

TO MAKE VEGETARIAN, OMIT THE CHICKEN, USE VEGETABLE BROTH INSTEAD OF BONE BROTH, AND SPRINKLE 3 TABLESPOONS NUTRITIONAL YEAST OVER THE FINISHED DISH.

3 tablespoons low-sodium chicken bone broth

¼ cup almond meal or almond flour

3 tablespoons coconut aminos

¼-inch piece fresh ginger, grated, or ½ teaspoon ground ginger

1 tablespoon avocado oil

1 cup ½-inch strips chicken breast

2 garlic cloves, minced

½ cup thinly sliced carrots

½ cup thinly sliced celery

3 cups broccoli florets

1 cup snow peas, fresh or thawed frozen

¼ cup cashews

2 cups cooked wild rice or quinoa

In a small saucepan, heat the bone broth over medium heat. Add the almond meal, coconut aminos, and ginger. Stir and let the mixture thicken slightly. Remove the pan from the heat and set aside.

In a large skillet, heat the oil over medium-high heat. Add the chicken and stir-fry for 5 minutes, or until no longer pink. Add the garlic, carrots, celery, broccoli, and snow peas and stir-fry for another 5 minutes or so, until tender. Add the broth mixture and cook for about 2 minutes more. Stir in the cashews.

Serve over the wild rice.

# SPRING SKILLET LASAGNA

SERVES 4 TO 6

TO MAKE VEGETARIAN, OMIT THE TURKEY AND SPRINKLE 1 TO 2 TABLESPOONS NUTRITIONAL YEAST OVER THE FINISHED DISH.

1 tablespoon avocado oil or extra-virgin olive oil

1 pound ground organic turkey

2 to 3 garlic cloves, to taste, minced

1 medium white onion, diced

1 bunch asparagus, ends trimmed, chopped into ½-inch pieces

2 zucchini, cut into ribbons or shredded

1 bunch baby spinach

1 cup frozen peas

2 Roma tomatoes, seeded and diced

1 teaspoon Italian seasoning

½ teaspoon dried oregano

Pinch of red pepper flakes

Sea salt and freshly ground black pepper

One 24-ounce jar clean marinara sauce (such as Rao's)

1 cup water

One 9-ounce box gluten-free lasagna noodles (such as Jovial), broken into pieces

¼ cup chopped fresh basil or parsley, for serving

We love to take traditional meals, like lasagna or a classic casserole, and amplify them to make them nutrient-dense and Feel-Good compliant. There is nothing wrong with continuing to enjoy your all-time favorite foods in their original form, but if you're looking for the Feel-Good change without giving up all your favorite meals, then you won't miss a thing from your traditional lasagna recipe with this version. We preserved the traditional flavor while adding in loads more fiber, greens, and various veggies.

In a large skillet, combine the oil, turkey, garlic, and onion and cook over medium heat, using a wooden spoon to break up the meat, until the turkey is cooked through, 8 to 10 minutes.

Add the asparagus, zucchini, spinach, peas, tomatoes, Italian seasoning, oregano, pepper flakes, and salt and black pepper to taste. Cook until the veggies are tender, about 5 minutes.

Add the marinara sauce, water, and broken lasagna noodles and stir well. Bring to a boil over medium-high heat, then reduce the heat to medium, cover, and cook, stirring often, until the lasagna noodles are just tender, about 15 minutes.

Sprinkle with the basil to serve.

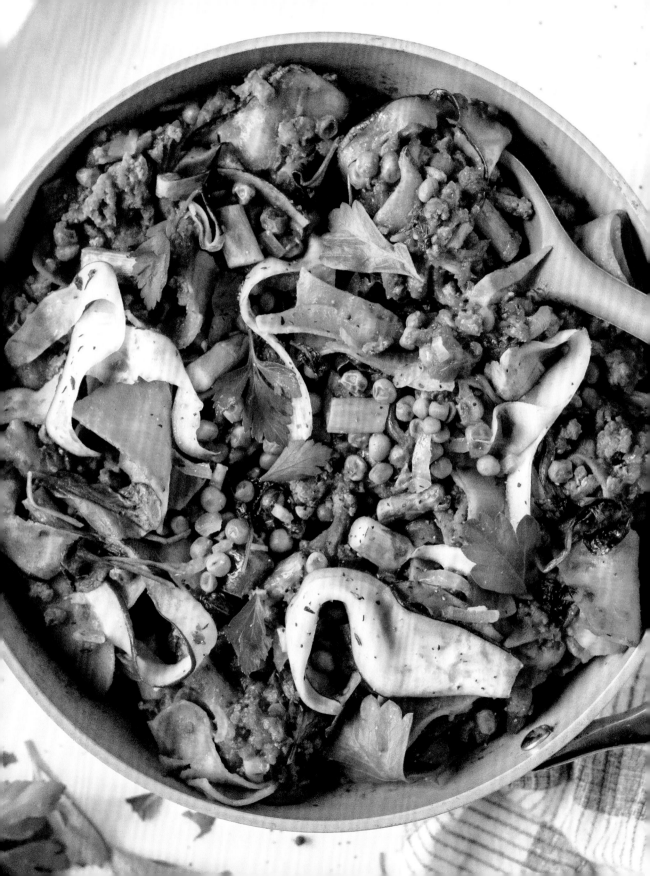

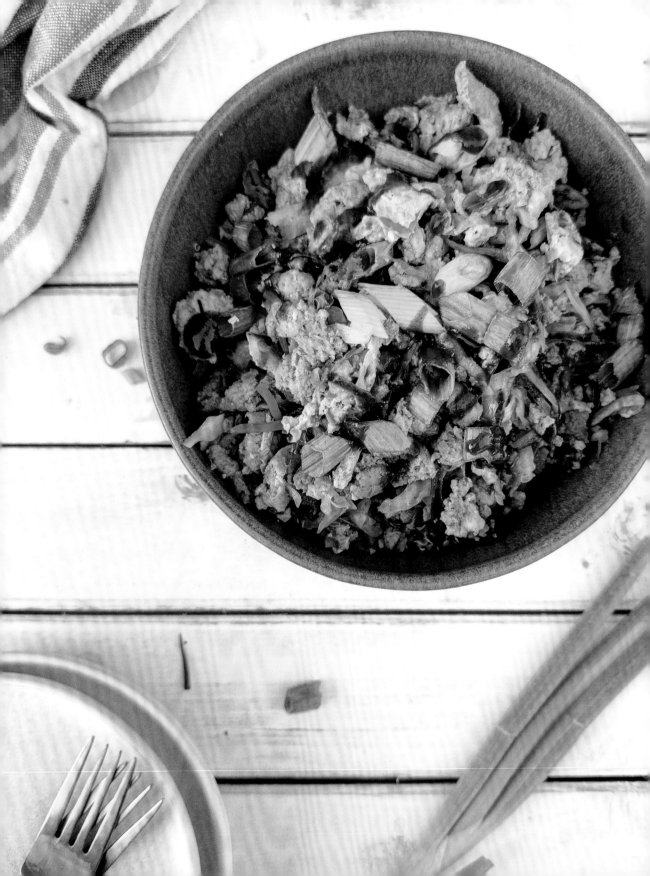

# EGG ROLL SKILLET

Another weeknight meal in one pan. Once you have some of the basic ingredients on hand, such as ginger and coconut aminos, these meals become even quicker and don't require too much thought. Have you tried coconut aminos yet? Coconut aminos taste similar to soy sauce. They are delicious, and I find sneaky ways to spruce up other meals with them. They run out a little faster than soy sauce might, because the flavor is much more subtle, and you may use more than your typical amount of soy sauce. You might want to go ahead and buy two bottles at a time.

**SERVES 4**
. . . . . . . . . . . . . . . . . . . . . . .
TO MAKE VEGETARIAN, OMIT THE CHICKEN OR TURKEY AND EGG AND ADD 4 TABLESPOONS NUTRITIONAL YEAST AFTER ADDING THE SRIRACHA.

1 tablespoon coconut oil

1 teaspoon minced garlic

1 pound ground organic chicken or turkey breast

14 ounces shredded cabbage or packaged coleslaw mix

¼ cup coconut aminos

1 teaspoon ground ginger

1 egg

2 teaspoons sriracha

2 cups cooked quinoa

1 tablespoon toasted sesame oil

2 tablespoons sliced green onions (optional)

In a large skillet, heat the coconut oil over medium heat. Add the garlic and sauté for 30 seconds. Add the chicken and cook until completely cooked through, 8 to 10 minutes.

Add the cabbage, coconut aminos, and ginger and sauté until the cabbage is tender, 5 to 7 minutes.

Make a well in the center of the skillet and add the egg. Scramble the egg over low heat until it's cooked through. Stir in the sriracha.

Divide the quinoa among four dishes. Top each serving of quinoa with one-quarter of the cabbage mixture. Drizzle with the sesame oil and more sriracha and sprinkle green onions (if using) on top.

# STUFFED PEPPERS

SERVES 6
. . . . . . . . . . . . . . . . . . . . . .
TO MAKE VEGETARIAN, OMIT
THE CHICKEN AND ADD
2 CUPS STEAMED LENTILS.

6 large bell peppers,
  halved lengthwise and
  cored (leave the stems
  intact, if you wish)

2 tablespoons extra-virgin
  olive oil, plus more for
  drizzling

Sea salt and freshly ground
  black pepper

1 white onion, finely diced

1 jalapeño chile (optional),
  minced

1 cup diced zucchini

1 cup diced yellow squash

1 cup fresh or frozen corn
  kernels

1 cup chopped cherry
  tomatoes

1 bunch green onions,
  thinly sliced

1 bunch fresh cilantro,
  roughly chopped

1 cup cooked quinoa

2 cups shredded organic
  rotisserie chicken

Fresh basil or chives
  (optional), finely
  chopped, for garnish

Lemon wedges (optional),
  for squeezing

*M*y husband is the pickiest person in our entire family, by far. He's also my most challenging client, I joke. He claims he doesn't like tomatoes and onions in his food or anything purple or anything that looks like fish eggs. The list goes on! BUT, this is one of those meals where I can actually make everyone happy, husband included! I stuff myself a few peppers and in the same pan, beside my peppers, I put the filling, or what I call the "slop," without the peppers. The whole family, even those who don't love peppers, can enjoy the same meal in different ways, which I'm a big fan of.

Preheat the oven to 475°F. Line a sheet pan with parchment paper or a silicone mat.

Place the bell peppers cut-side down on the lined pan. Drizzle with some oil. Season with salt and black pepper.

Transfer to the oven and roast until the peppers begin to blister, 15 to 20 minutes.

Remove the pan from the oven and turn the peppers over. Set aside. Leave the oven on.

Meanwhile, in a large skillet, heat the 2 tablespoons olive oil over high heat. Add the onion and jalapeño (if using). Reduce the heat to medium and season with salt and black pepper. Cook, stirring occasionally, until the onion is softened and translucent, about 5 minutes.

Add the zucchini and squash and cook until just crisp-tender, about 2 minutes. Add the corn and cook for a minute more. Remove the skillet from the heat. Add the tomatoes, green onions, cilantro, quinoa, and chicken. Season with salt and black pepper.

Spoon the mixture from the skillet into the peppers until they are heaping, nearly overfilled. (If you have extra filling, save it to eat on its own, topped on a salad, or added to over easy or scrambled eggs.)

Return the pan of peppers to the oven and cook for 10 minutes, until they can be easily punctured with a fork.

If desired, serve the peppers garnished with fresh basil and with a fresh lemon wedge to squeeze over the top.

# PLANTAIN-CRUSTED "FRIED" CHICKEN WITH MASHED SWEET POTATOES

*I* usually reserve this recipe for a slower evening, or even a Sunday afternoon, since it is a little more in-depth. It's well worth your time and effort. And the mashed sweet potatoes will rock your food world! Anything whipped is up my alley. I love soft, fluffy, and creamy. I hope you enjoy this one as much as my family does!

## SERVES 4

### MASHED SWEET POTATOES

2 pounds sweet potatoes, scrubbed

¼ cup canned full-fat coconut milk, plus more as needed

½ teaspoon ground cinnamon

Sea salt and freshly ground black pepper

### "FRIED" CHICKEN

One 4-ounce bag plantain chips made with clean ingredients and cooked in coconut oil (such as Barnana or Terra) or homemade Plantain Chips (page 136)

¼ teaspoon sea salt

½ teaspoon garlic powder

½ teaspoon onion powder

1 teaspoon smoked paprika

½ teaspoon dried oregano

¼ cup coconut oil

1 pound organic chicken tenders

½ cup steamed broccoli, for serving

Preheat the oven to 400°F. Line a baking sheet with parchment paper or a silicone baking mat.

To make the mashed sweet potatoes: Using a fork, prick the sweet potatoes in a few spots, then place them on the lined baking sheet.

Bake until tender, 45 minutes to 1 hour, depending on their size. Remove the sweet potatoes from the oven and set aside to cool. Leave the oven on.

When the sweet potatoes are cool enough to handle, peel them and move them to a medium pot. Set the pot over medium-low heat and mash the peeled sweet potatoes with a potato masher. Add the coconut milk as you mash, starting with ¼ cup, then adding more as needed. Season the mashed sweet potatoes with the cinnamon and salt and pepper to taste.

To make the "fried" chicken: In a food processor, pulse the plantain chips for 30 to 60 seconds, or until ground into a "breading" texture, being sure not to grind the chips too finely, as you want the chicken strips to have some crunch.

Transfer the plantain chip breading to a medium shallow bowl. Stir in the salt, garlic powder, onion powder, smoked paprika, and oregano until well combined. Add the coconut oil to a small shallow bowl.

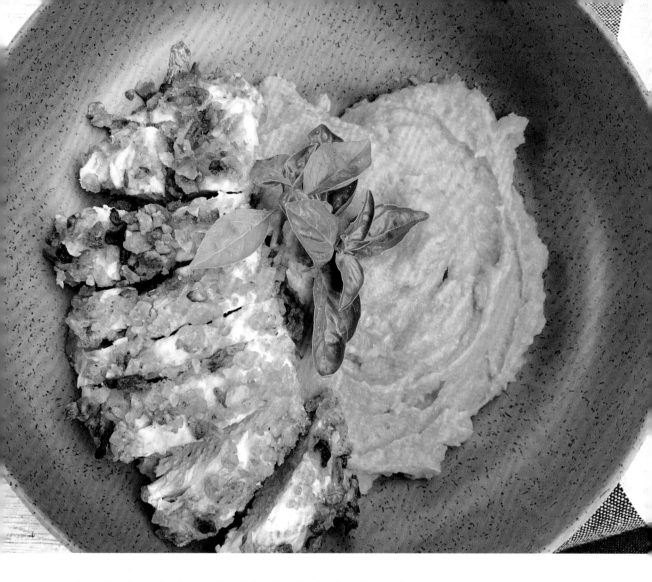

One at a time, dredge each chicken tender in the oil, gently shaking off any excess. Then place in the bowl of plantain chip breading and coat both sides. Arrange them on a baking sheet lined with parchment paper.

Bake for 20 minutes. Flip and bake until crispy, an additional 10 to 15 minutes.

To serve, divide the potatoes among four plates and place the chicken strips on top or alongside the potatoes. Serve broccoli on the side to add more colors.

# *Heather*

Heather came to CCN after the pandemic. Over the last couple of years, she noticed she had gained some weight and lapsed into unhealthy habits. (Sound familiar, anybody?) She was not sure she wanted to start another diet, but she really wanted to lose some weight.

It took her only two weeks of following the Feel-Good Way philosophy to appreciate the change in her lifestyle. She described the experience as finding herself again. She felt not only more energetic but also more optimistic and positive during her daily interactions with other people—most especially with her children. Now that she had a plan for what to cook for dinner and knew it would be healthy and taste good, she made it a priority for the family to sit down at the table together as many nights of the week as possible. This one shift in the family dynamic changed everything.

As a mother of four, she'd become accustomed to feeling overwhelmed pretty much all the time. Just keeping her head above water was a constant struggle. Looking after herself came last in her long list of responsibilities and worries. But when she began getting healthy, following the Feel-Good fundamentals and providing healthy choices for her family, she found a new purpose, and she started to see the bigger picture. After she created a standard of feeling good in her home, her life began to change. She'd assumed it would be difficult to do something new, to make changes. In hindsight, she saw that the healthier way was much easier than trying to keep up how she'd been just getting by before.

There aren't a lot of diets out there that talk about mood or family dynamics—and why would they, some might ask. But I truly believe in the connection between what we put into our bodies and how it makes us feel. That connection can lead to better relationships with ourselves and others—not to mention our faith. As we feel better, not only is our body lighter, our mind is clearer. We become more excited and energized to grow inward. We experience the opening of a new world of possibility with our faith and the energy we now have to dedicate to more prayer, to serving others, to finding our greater purpose—or simply to being confident that we are doing exactly what we are supposed to be doing.

# SLOW COOKER VEGGIE BAKED PENNE

*D*ump it, forget it, then enjoy it! That's all you have to know with this dish. So good and so easy to make. We all need dishes in our rotation that we don't have to think about. As a mom, I know one of the things that can weigh me down mentally is all the planning that goes into a typical day—especially meal planning. One of my favorite things about my job is taking that load off parents having to constantly decide what to make for dinner that is healthy and that everyone will like. So let me help you: Add this one to your go-to list.

**SERVES 6**

**VEGETARIAN**

Avocado or coconut oil cooking spray

One 15-ounce container 2% milkfat cottage cheese

2 eggs

⅓ cup chopped fresh basil, plus more for garnish

Two 25-ounce jars clean marinara sauce (such as Rao's)

1 pound uncooked whole-grain penne pasta (such as whole wheat, brown rice, quinoa, etc.)

1 medium zucchini, diced

2 cups freshly grated Parmesan or Romano cheese

1 medium yellow squash, diced

½ cup grated Asiago cheese

Red pepper flakes (optional), for serving

Coat the inside of the slow cooker with cooking spray. In a large bowl, combine the cottage cheese, eggs, and basil and stir well.

Add 2 cups of the marinara sauce to the bottom of the slow cooker. Add one-third of the penne, then layer with half of the cottage cheese mixture, spreading it over the top. Add the diced zucchini and sprinkle with half of the Parmesan. Repeat the layers, using yellow squash instead of zucchini. Add the last of the penne and top it with the remaining sauce.

Cover and cook on high for 3½ to 4 hours, or until the pasta is cooked through. During the last few minutes of cooking, sprinkle the Asiago over the top and let it melt.

Divide the penne among bowls and sprinkle with basil and pepper flakes (if using).

# SALSA VERDE SMOTHERED BURRITOS

**SERVES 4 TO 6**

TO MAKE VEGETARIAN, OMIT THE BEEF.

1 teaspoon extra-virgin olive oil or avocado oil

1 small yellow onion, minced

1 garlic clove, minced

1 pound grass-fed ground beef

1 cup frozen cauliflower rice

1½ cups fresh spinach leaves (or frozen, but be sure to thaw and drain first)

One 1-ounce packet clean taco seasoning (such as Siete), or 2 tablespoons Homemade Taco Seasoning (page 189)

Juice of 1 lime

1 cup canned organic black beans

Sea salt and freshly ground black pepper

4 to 6 gluten-free burrito-size tortillas (such as Siete)

Handful of fresh cilantro, chopped

One 16-ounce jar salsa verde (look for a brand that is clean with a short ingredients list)

**FOR SERVING**

1 avocado, sliced

Fresh cilantro

*T*his is another weeknight meal that hopefully the whole family will love, but here is one of my secrets to life: If your family doesn't love the meal as much as you do, then you get more leftovers for yourself at lunch the next day. And if your family *does* love the meal as much as you do, then you can all enjoy the meal together. Either way, you're winning. Back to the burritos, though—I don't think you'll have to worry about anyone not liking these!

Preheat the oven to 350°F. Line a shallow baking dish with parchment paper.

In a large skillet, heat the oil over medium heat. When the oil is hot and starting to make popping noises, add the onion and garlic and sauté for 5 minutes. Add the meat, stirring to combine, and cook until no longer pink, 8 to 10 minutes.

Add the cauliflower and spinach and sauté for another 5 minutes, until the spinach is wilted. Mix in the taco seasoning and half of the lime juice. Remove the pan from the heat, transfer the meat/veggie mixture to a large bowl, and set aside.

In a medium bowl, combine the black beans and the remaining lime juice. Using the back of a fork, mash the beans so that they form a nice paste. Season with salt and pepper and set aside.

Heat the skillet over medium heat again. Place a tortilla in the pan for about 15 seconds per side. (Alternatively, you can microwave the tortillas for about 15 seconds.) Heating the tortillas helps to make them more flexible and less likely to tear. Set the tortillas on a plate or board to assemble.

Dividing the ingredients evenly among the tortillas, on the middle of each tortilla layer the bean mixture, meat/veggie mixture, and cilantro. Fold the bottom of the tortilla up and over the filling, then fold the two sides over the filling, creating an envelope with the filling in the center. Roll the top flap of the burrito tightly over the filling until fully rolled up.

Put each completed burrito in the baking dish, seam-side down. Cover the burritos with half of the salsa verde, spreading it evenly over the burritos.

Bake for 15 minutes to warm through. Serve with the remaining salsa and the avocado and cilantro.

# SALT AND VINEGAR FISH 'N' CHIPS

SERVES 4

**TARTAR SAUCE**

½ cup coconut or avocado oil mayo (such as Primal Kitchen, Chosen Foods, or Sir Kensington)

1½ tablespoons Frank's RedHot sauce (or your preferred brand)

1 teaspoon apple cider vinegar

1 dill pickle, finely diced

**POTATOES**

1½ pounds baby potatoes, chopped

1 cup distilled white vinegar

2 garlic cloves, smashed

1 tablespoon sea salt

**FISH**

1 egg, lightly beaten

½ cup almond flour

1 teaspoon garlic powder

1 teaspoon onion powder

Sea salt and freshly ground black pepper

4 fillets wild-caught cod (3 to 4 ounces each), or other firm white fish (such as mahimahi), thawed if previously frozen

1 tablespoon ghee or coconut oil

*F*ish 'n' chips always makes me think of a restaurant on the water. From Lake Michigan to the Pacific to the Gulf in Florida, there is nothing like a fresh order of fish and chips. Go there in your mind with this recipe, without the weighted-down feeling you get after leaving a restaurant. This recipe calls for cod, but freshwater fish such as perch, walleye, and trout also work well if you're near the Great Lakes with a fresh catch! Or try any firm white fish. Just make sure it's a thick fillet so that it doesn't fall apart during cooking.

To make the tartar sauce: In a small bowl, combine the mayo, hot sauce, vinegar, and pickle and mix well. The sauce can be made beforehand and stored in the fridge a few days ahead of time if desired.

To cook the potatoes: Preheat the oven to 425°F. Line a large baking sheet with parchment paper.

In a large pot, combine the chopped potatoes and vinegar and add cold water until the potatoes are submerged. Bring the pot to a boil, then add the garlic and salt and cook the potatoes until fork-tender, about 20 minutes.

Meanwhile, to prepare the fish: Place the egg in a shallow bowl. In another shallow bowl, combine the almond flour, garlic powder, and onion powder and season to taste with salt and pepper.

Pat the fish dry with a paper towel. Dip each fillet in the egg wash, then dredge it in the almond flour mixture until evenly coated.

In a large skillet, heat the ghee over low heat. Add the fish and cook until browned on both sides, about 2 minutes per side. Remove the fillets from the pan and set aside.

2 tablespoons avocado oil

1½ teaspoons sea salt

To finish: Drain the cooked potatoes and spread them on the parchment-lined baking sheet. If needed, use two baking sheets to ensure enough space between the potatoes. Drizzle the avocado oil over the potatoes and sprinkle with the salt. Toss the potatoes until evenly coated.

Bake the potatoes for 15 minutes.

Take the potatoes out of the oven and flip. Reduce the oven temperature to 400°F. Place the fish in the middle of the pan, arranging the potatoes around the outside.

Return to the oven and bake until the fish flakes easily with a fork and the potatoes are golden brown and crispy, an additional 10 to 15 minutes.

# CHILI LIME CHICKEN

CHILI LIME CHICKEN

6 boneless, skinless
   chicken thighs, or
   4 boneless, skinless
   chicken breasts

2 limes

4 garlic cloves, minced

3 tablespoons extra-virgin
   olive oil

1 teaspoon chili powder

1 to 2 teaspoons red
   pepper flakes

Sea salt and freshly ground
   black pepper

1 tablespoon homemade
   Chili Seasoning (recipe
   follows) or store-bought
   chile-lime seasoning
   (such as Trader Joe's)

ASSEMBLY

2 tablespoons avocado oil

1 cup uncooked brown rice

One 16-ounce bag frozen
   broccoli

2½ cups chicken or beef
   bone broth or vegetable
   broth

Juice of 1 lime, plus a
   squeeze

1 tablespoon plus
   ¼ teaspoon homemade
   Chili Seasoning or
   store-bought chile-lime
   seasoning (such as
   Trader Joe's)

Chopped fresh cilantro, for
   serving

*H*ere's another meal my girls request on the regular. The
flavor is somehow bold and subtle at the same time. My
girls enjoy zesty flavors, like lime and balsamic vinegar, maybe
more than most. If you aren't a tangy, citrus-loving family, this
may not end up in your rotation, but I hope it does, because it
makes a great weeknight meal.

To marinate the chicken: With a rolling pin or meat pounder,
pound the chicken to an even thickness.

Use a zester to grate the zest of one of the limes. Then juice
both limes, saving the spent rinds. In a small bowl, combine
the zest, juice, garlic, olive oil, and chili powder. Season with
red pepper flakes, salt, and black pepper to taste. Whisk together. Add the lime rinds.

Place the chicken in a baking dish, add the marinade, and
toss to coat and baste. Marinate for 2 hours in the fridge.

Remove the chicken from the marinade and discard the
marinade. Season the chicken with the chili seasoning and
more salt and black pepper to taste.

To assemble the dish: Drizzle a large skillet with the oil and
heat over medium heat. Add the chicken to the skillet and
cook until browned on both sides, 3 to 4 minutes per side.
Remove the chicken from the pan.

Add the rice, broccoli, broth, lime juice, and chili seasoning
to the skillet. Set the chicken on top of the rice and broccoli,
cover, and cook until the liquid is absorbed, 20 to 25 minutes.

Fluff the rice with a fork and top with cilantro and one more
squeeze of lime.

*(continues on page 212)*

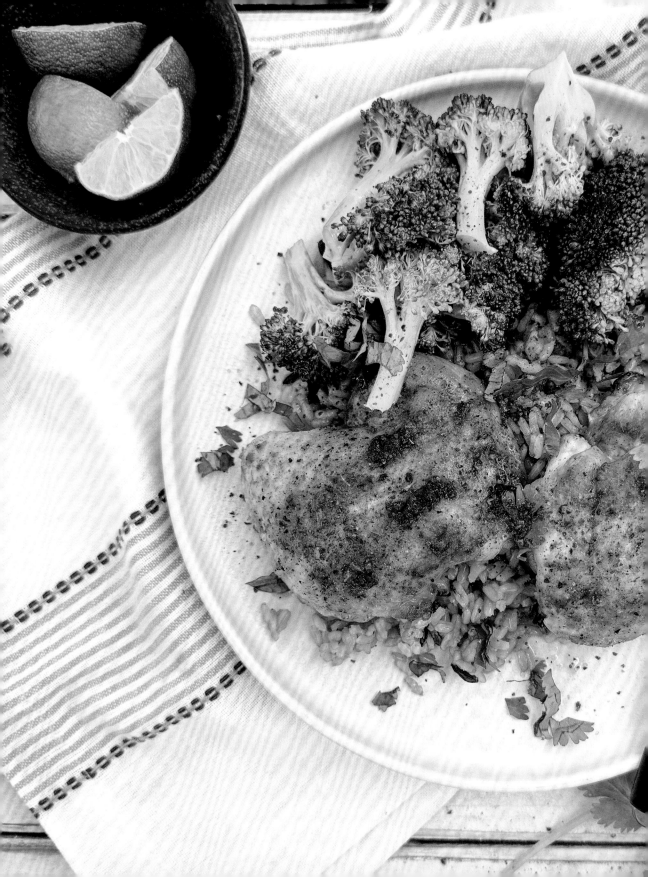

· · · · · · · · · · · · · · · · · · · · · · ·

¼ cup chili powder

1½ tablespoons paprika

1½ tablespoons garlic
     powder

1½ tablespoons onion
     powder

1 teaspoon cayenne pepper

## CHILI SEASONING

In a small bowl, whisk together all the ingredients to combine. Transfer to an airtight container.

# BLACKENED SHRIMP KEBABS

*T*hese kebabs are perfect for summer nights when nobody wants to heat the house with the oven. They cook so perfectly on the grill. While the peach salsa is delicious and helps to improve the carb count for this meal, you could instead serve the kebabs over a bowl of rice or quinoa with a big green salad on the side. Surprise your friends and neighbors with these at the next barbecue! They'll be asking for the recipe for sure.

**SERVES 4**

1½ pounds jumbo or extra-large shrimp, peeled and deveined

2 tablespoons Blackening Spice (recipe follows)

Avocado oil

Peach Salsa (recipe follows)

Preheat the grill to medium-high heat.

Wash and pat dry the shrimp. Thread the shrimp onto skewers, about 4 per skewer. Season with the blackening spice and drizzle with avocado oil.

Place the shrimp on the grill and cook for 2 to 3 minutes on each side. Serve with the peach salsa.

2 tablespoons garlic powder

2 tablespoons chili powder

1 tablespoon ground cumin

1 tablespoon paprika

2 teaspoons cayenne pepper

1 teaspoon sea salt

## BLACKENING SPICE

**MAKES 7 TABLESPOONS**

In a small bowl, combine all the ingredients and mix well. Transfer to an airtight container.

1 plum tomato, seeded and roughly chopped

½ jalapeño chile, seeded

½ small red onion, roughly chopped

¼ cup chopped fresh cilantro

3 peaches, peeled and chopped, pits removed

Sea salt and freshly ground black pepper

## PEACH SALSA

**MAKES 1 CUP**

In a food processor, combine the tomato, jalapeño, red onion, and cilantro. Pulse to roughly chop. Mix in the peaches by hand and season to taste with salt and pepper.

# SALMON SHEET PAN

SERVES 4
. . . . . . . . . . . . . . . . . . . . . . .
TO MAKE VEGETARIAN, USE
1 CUP CHICKPEAS IN PLACE
OF THE SALMON, THEN
SPRINKLE WITH ¼ CUP SEEDS,
SUCH AS SUNFLOWER,
PUMPKIN, OR HEMP.

Avocado or coconut oil
    cooking spray

4 wild-caught salmon
    fillets (4 to 6 ounces
    each)

1 lemon, half sliced and
    half left for squeezing

1 bunch asparagus (about
    1 pound), ends trimmed

4 thin slices red onion,
    quartered

3 garlic cloves, sliced

5 radishes, sliced

1 pint grape tomatoes,
    halved

Himalayan pink salt and
    freshly ground black
    pepper

Extra-virgin olive oil (try a
    flavor-infused variety—
    garlic is great!)

2 cups cooked quinoa or
    wild rice, for serving

Chopped fresh basil
    (optional), for garnish

*L*ike so many of you, I get bogged down with dirty dishes from time to time. I tend to cook no less than three times a day because I personally don't love eating out. Occasionally my kids aren't too busy to help with the evening dishes, but when they are, I find myself wanting one-pan or sheet-pan dinners. That way we're not depriving ourselves of flavor and taste and we're not spending hours in the kitchen afterward. This salmon sheet pan dinner is one of those meals that give us all what we want. If you and your family don't eat fish, you could try chicken or sausage in its place.

Preheat the oven to broil. Coat a large sheet pan with cooking spray.

Put the salmon fillets in the center of the pan and top with the lemon slices. Surround the salmon on all sides with the asparagus. Sprinkle red onion and garlic over the top, then top with radishes and tomatoes. Season everything with salt and pepper. Lightly drizzle with olive oil. Squeeze the remaining lemon over everything.

Broil until the salmon is cooked through and the veggies are crisp-tender, 10 to 15 minutes.

Serve over quinoa and garnish with basil if desired.

# SPICY LETTUCE WRAPS

SERVES 6 TO 8

TO MAKE VEGETARIAN, SUBSTITUTE ONE 15-OUNCE CAN ORGANIC BLACK BEANS OR CHICKPEAS FOR THE CHICKEN AND TOP THE WRAPS WITH YOUR CHOICE OF NUTS OR SEEDS.

1 pound boneless, skinless chicken breasts

½ cup chicken or bone broth or vegetable broth

¾ cup clean Buffalo sauce (such as Primal Kitchen)

½ cup 2% plain Greek yogurt

2 medium carrots, shredded

2 celery stalks, chopped

2 garlic cloves, minced

½ medium white or yellow onion, chopped

Sea salt and freshly ground black pepper

ASSEMBLY

Lettuce cups (head of Bibb, Boston, or romaine lettuce)

Shredded carrot

Finely chopped celery

Blue or feta cheese crumbles

Chopped green onion

Avocado slices

3 to 4 cups cooked rice (¾ cup per serving)

My kids always ask me why we only make these lettuce wraps when we have guests. I don't think that's totally true, but for some reason these are my go-to when we have people coming over. I make them with the intention of having plenty of leftovers to serve the next day, but no matter how much I make, we almost never have leftovers. My family loves them that much! Sometimes my girls forget about the rice altogether because they get so full on the wraps! I hope this will be a hit in your home as well.

In a slow cooker, combine the chicken, chicken broth, ½ cup of the Buffalo sauce, the yogurt, carrots, celery, garlic, and onion. Season with salt and pepper. Cover and cook on low for 7 to 8 hours or high for 4 to 5 hours, stirring a few times through the cooking process to keep the chicken coated with sauce.

Drain the excess liquid from the slow cooker and shred the chicken with two forks. (You can also use a stand mixer fitted with the paddle.)

Add the remaining ¼ cup Buffalo sauce to the shredded chicken and toss to coat. Return the chicken to the slow cooker and cook on high for 30 minutes before serving.

To assemble the lettuce wraps: Lay out the lettuce cups and top each with the Buffalo chicken mixture. Add the shredded carrot, celery, a sprinkle of blue or feta cheese, green onion, and avocado. Serve with rice on the side.

# THAI CAULIFLOWER PIZZA

*H*ave you heard the saying "If cauliflower can be pizza, then you, my friend, can be anything"? I'm not a fan of cauliflower *everything,* but this pizza is so good, you won't even realize you're missing traditional pizza crust. And the Thai flair will excite your taste buds and have you adding this meal to your regular rotation. If you eat the whole thing yourself, just know I've been there and done that before!

**SERVES 4**

VEGETARIAN

⅓ cup Peanut Sauce (recipe follows), plus more for drizzling

1 prepared cauliflower pizza crust (such as Trader Joe's or CauliPower)

1 cup canned organic chickpeas, rinsed and drained

1 bell pepper, thinly sliced

2 carrots, shaved or shredded

2 green onions, chopped

Fresh cilantro, for garnish

Bean sprouts or microgreens (optional), for garnish

Preheat the oven to 375°F.

Spread the ⅓ cup peanut sauce over the crust. Top with the chickpeas, bell pepper, carrots, and green onions.

Bake the pizza until all the ingredients are heated through, 10 to 12 minutes.

Drizzle 1 to 2 tablespoons of peanut sauce on top of the pizza. Garnish with the cilantro and sprouts (if using) before serving.

**PEANUT SAUCE**

MAKES ABOUT 1⅓ CUPS

½ cup natural peanut butter

2 tablespoons toasted sesame oil

¼ cup coconut aminos

¼ cup water

1 tablespoon sriracha

½-inch slice fresh ginger, minced

2 garlic cloves, minced

In a food processor or blender, combine the peanut butter, sesame oil, coconut aminos, water, sriracha, ginger, and garlic and process until smooth. Add a little more water if needed. Use right away or store in an airtight container for up to 1 week.

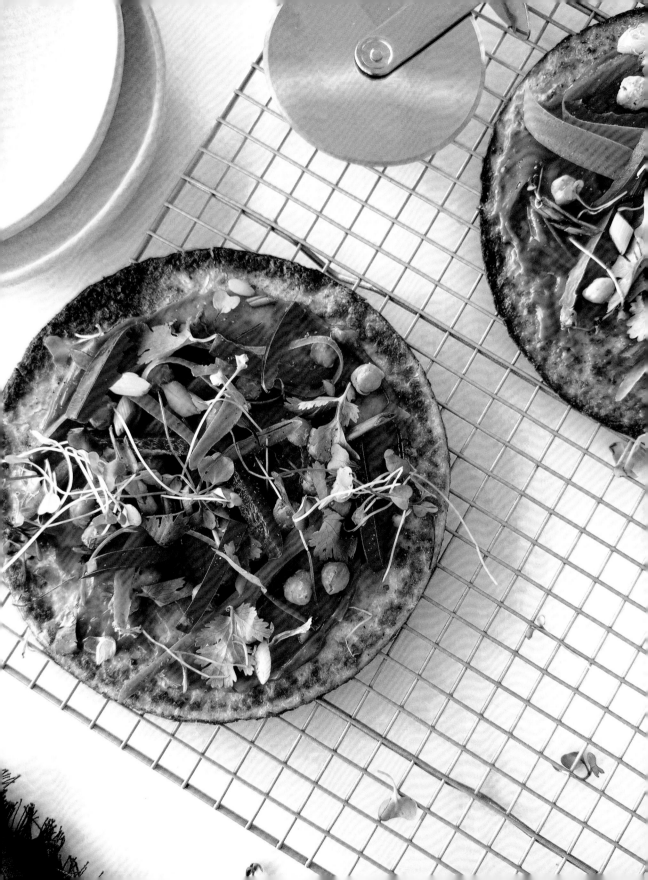

# FISH TACO SLAW BOWLS

*F*ish tacos are always my beach vacation go-to. But even when we're eating at restaurants, I tend to turn the tacos into a bowl. I don't personally need double corn tortillas wrapping fresh fish, cabbage, and a delicious sauce, so I usually get a small side salad, eat one taco as is, and then dump the rest into the bowl. Why not create that very favorite vacation meal right in a bowl? (If you don't want to skip the tacos, you can still add taco shells and fill them with the ingredients. In that case, I'd skip the rice.)

**SERVES 4**

TO MAKE VEGETARIAN, OMIT THE FISH AND SUBSTITUTE ½ CUP CANNED ORGANIC PINTO BEANS OR AN ADDITIONAL ½ CUP BLACK BEANS INSTEAD.

4 pieces wild-caught white fish (4 to 6 ounces each), such as cod, grouper, or sole

1 tablespoon avocado oil

1 tablespoon Homemade Taco Seasoning (page 189)

½ cup thinly sliced green onion

One 14-ounce bag coleslaw mix

½ medium head red cabbage, shredded

Spicy Lime Aioli (recipe follows)

**FOR SERVING**

1 cup cooked black beans

1 cup cooked brown rice or quinoa (optional)

Salsa or pico de gallo

Guacamole

Fresh cilantro

Lime wedges

Drizzle the fish with 1½ teaspoons of the avocado oil and rub with the taco seasoning.

Brush a grill pan or skillet with the remaining 1½ teaspoons oil and heat the pan over medium-high heat. Add the fish and cook for 4 minutes. Flip and cook until the fish is barely firm and flakes easily with a fork, another 3 to 4 minutes, depending on the thickness of your fish.

Meanwhile, in a large bowl, combine half of the green onions with the coleslaw and shredded cabbage and mix. Stir in just enough of the spicy lime aioli to barely moisten the cabbage.

When the fish is done, let it cool slightly on a cutting board, then use two forks to shred the fish.

To serve: Fill four bowls each with one-quarter of the slaw mixture and top with the fish. Drizzle a little more aioli over the top. Add the beans, rice (if using), salsa, a dollop of guacamole, some cilantro, the remaining green onions, and a lime wedge to each bowl. Serve immediately.

**NOTE:** To avoid the smell of fish inside your house, opt for an outside grill or broil the fish for 4 to 6 minutes.

**SPICY LIME AIOLI**

In a small bowl, whisk together the mayo, lime zest, lime juice, hot sauce, and salt to taste.

½ cup coconut or avocado oil mayo

½ teaspoon grated lime zest

2 tablespoons fresh lime juice

2 teaspoons hot sauce

Sea salt

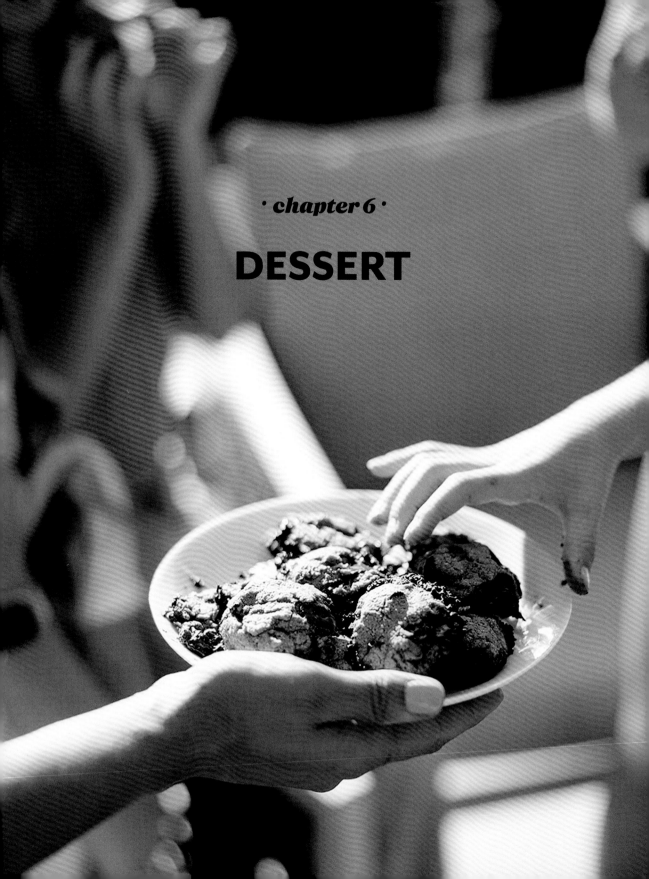

· chapter 6 ·

# DESSERT

......................

**The dessert recipes** in this chapter don't need to be considered a special treat. They are nutrient-rich and energy-dense. They add value—not guilt—to your daily diet!

I've met so many people who fear carbs and think dessert must go out the window when they start trying to make healthier choices. Over time, the emotional toll of those choices can weigh heavier on them than the carbs themselves. It's important that food be enjoyed and not worried about or regretted. If I choose to have a dessert at the end of the day, it's for the enjoyment and nourishment of my body and soul, not guilt or fear.

These recipes deliver what our bodies need and allow us to enjoy a wholesome sweetness. When you eat these healthful desserts, you won't experience the tired, blah feelings you may normally have after dessert. Instead, you're likely to feel satisfied and realize how easy it is to stay committed to your own health. As with the snacks, any of these desserts can be eaten as a meal themselves. These recipes are loaded with minerals, antioxidants, vitamins, enzymes, and more.

Here's a blessing that grounds eating a healthy, delicious dessert as a gift instead of something to fear or cause emotional shame or anxiety.

**Bless this** dessert to satiate my craving and provide pleasure to my taste buds. Bless the foods that were used to prepare this delicious treat to nourish my body in the depth of my cells. Bless the hands, especially if they were my own, that prepared this dessert to be attuned to health on the deepest level. I bind up any fear that could cause emotional or mental distress when enjoying the pleasure of foods that are able to provide my body the nutrients it needs. Allow me to enjoy and utilize these foods in their fullness, dear God. In your name, we pray. Amen.

# FUDGE BROWNIES

*I* try really hard not to say that every recipe is my favorite ever, but for this book I really have pulled together my all-time favorite recipes. For example, I absolutely love these fudge brownies. They are perfectly rich and chewy, and most people would probably guess they're from a box. They're so good! Fair warning . . . these brownies are so high in fiber, they may send you for an extra potty break!

**SERVES 12**

5 ounces dark chocolate or chocolate chips

¼ cup coconut oil

3 eggs, at room temperature

¾ cup coconut sugar

1 cup almond flour or flaxseed meal

⅓ cup cacao powder

Pinch of sea salt

Preheat the oven to 350°F. Line an 8 by 8-inch baking pan with parchment paper.

In a double boiler (or in a pot or bowl placed on top of a pot with two inches of water set to boil), melt the chocolate and coconut oil together, stirring to combine. Set aside.

In a medium bowl, with an electric mixer, combine the eggs and coconut sugar and beat until smooth and fluffy. Add the melted chocolate and beat for another minute. Add the almond flour, cacao powder, and salt. Gently fold together until the batter is smooth.

Pour the batter into the prepared baking pan and bake until a toothpick inserted in the center comes out clean, about 18 minutes.

Serve warm or cool. Store in a closed container in the fridge for up to 4 days.

# CHOCOLATE PB BARS

*T*his is another quick and easy recipe that my kids and friends regularly request. These give the same vibe and taste as a traditional chewy bar, but they're packed with ingredients that make us feel good, too. Make sure to leave some time for chilling if you're going to cut the bars into neat squares and serve. Otherwise, they get super messy. Another thing to remember is that all the nut butters and seed butters are interchangeable. If you have food allergies in your home, swap the nut butter with whatever works for you.

**MAKES 10 TO 12 BARS**

**VEGETARIAN**

1½ cups natural peanut butter

½ cup raw or mānuka honey

⅓ cup virgin coconut oil

1½ cups oat flour

¼ cup flaxseed meal (optional)

1½ cups semisweet chocolate chips

Line a 9 by 9-inch square baking pan with parchment paper.

In a large bowl, combine the peanut butter, honey, and coconut oil and mix. Add the oat flour and flaxseed meal (if using) and stir until well combined. The mixture will be thick.

Press the mixture evenly into the prepared baking pan.

In a microwave-safe bowl, melt the chocolate chips in the microwave in 20- to 30-second intervals, stirring after each. (Alternatively, melt them on the stove using a double boiler.) Stir the melted chips until smooth. Pour the chocolate sauce evenly over the peanut butter bars. Smooth with the back of a spoon or rubber spatula.

Chill in the refrigerator for about 2 hours. Let it sit at room temperature for 10 minutes before cutting into bars. Keep refrigerated or freeze.

# GLUTEN-FREE CHEWY CHOCOLATE CHUNK COOKIES

*I*f you're new to coconut sugar, you might be wondering why these chocolate chip cookies call for coconut sugar instead of natural cane sugar. The two are actually pretty interchangeable, but coconut sugar contains essential minerals, vitamins, antioxidants, and fiber that other sugar options do not offer.

**MAKES 24 COOKIES**

VEGETARIAN IF YOU USE
A FLAX/CHIA EGG (SEE
PAGE 39).

1 cup superfine almond
   flour

¼ cup coconut flour

¼ teaspoon ground
   cinnamon

1 teaspoon baking soda

6 tablespoons grass-
   fed butter, at room
   temperature

¾ cup packed coconut
   sugar

¼ cup plus 2 tablespoons
   natural almond,
   cashew, or other nut/
   seed butter

1 egg, at room temperature

1½ teaspoons pure vanilla
   extract

1¼ cups chocolate chunks
   or chips (70% or more
   cocoa)

Preheat the oven to 350°F. Line a baking sheet with parchment paper or a silicone mat.

In a medium bowl, combine the almond flour, coconut flour, cinnamon, and baking soda and whisk together. Set aside.

In a stand mixer fitted with the paddle, beat the butter, coconut sugar, and almond butter on medium speed for 2 minutes. Scrape down the sides if needed. Add the egg and vanilla and beat on low until well mixed. Add the flour mixture and beat on low until well combined. Fold in 1 cup of the chocolate chunks.

Using a cookie scoop, spoon, or your hands, drop 2-inch balls of the cookie dough onto the prepared baking sheet. Gently press down with your hands to spread the dough a bit. Top with the reserved chocolate chunks and gently press them in.

Bake until the edges are lightly golden brown, 11 to 14 minutes.

Let the cookies cool for 5 minutes on the pan, then transfer to a wire rack to cool completely.

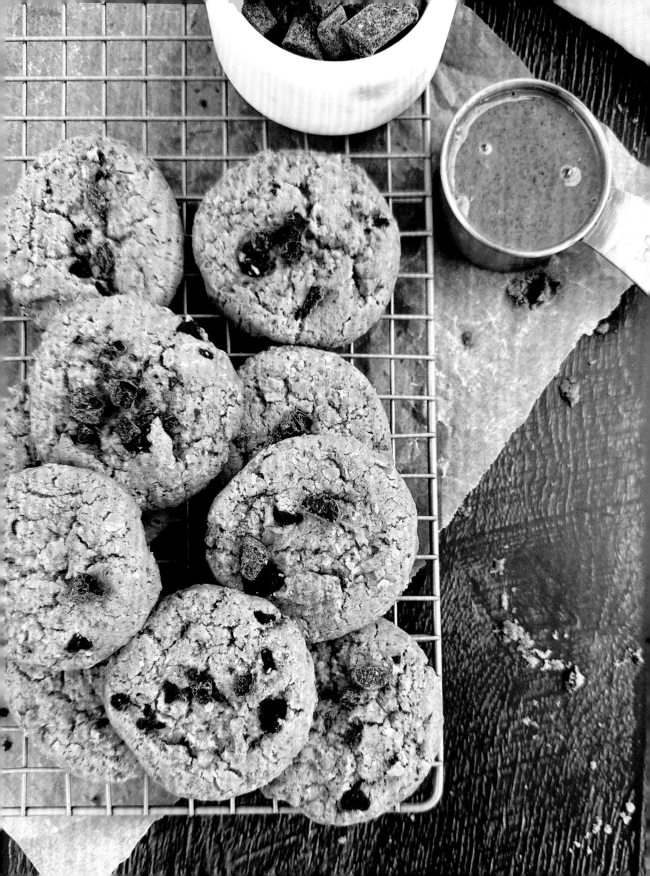

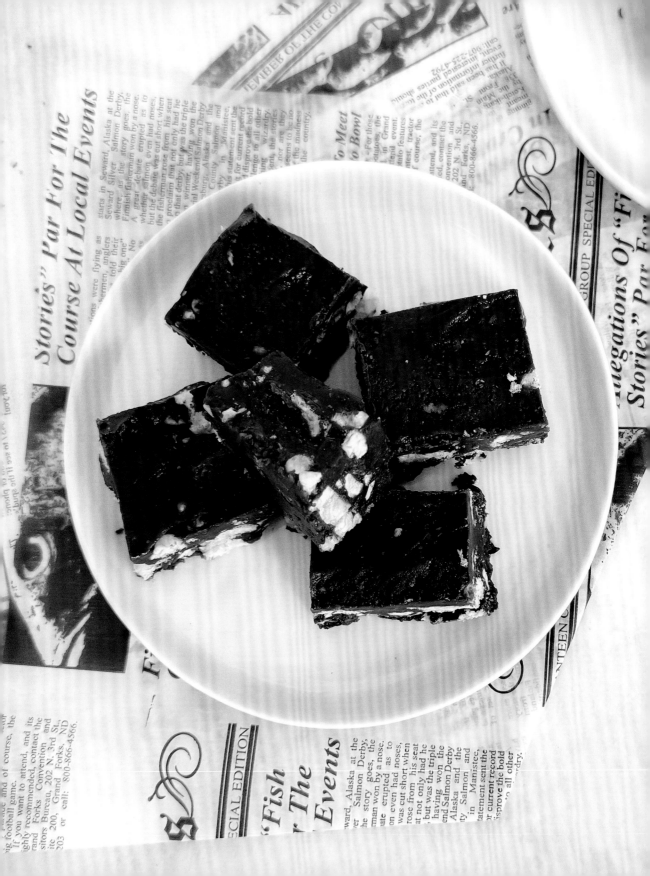

# CHOCOLATE KRISPIE TREATS

When my girls have weeknight sports practice, they come home around 9:00 P.M. completely famished, as though I hadn't fed them dinner beforehand! They usually want something sweet, and these no-bake treats have become a go-to. A no-bake treat is also the perfect opportunity to work in honey. Honey has so many health benefits, but we aren't likely to receive them if the honey has been heated, as studies have shown honey loses its antibacterial properties under high heat.

**MAKES 9 SQUARES
(SERVES 2 OR 3)**
. . . . . . . . . . . . . . . . . . . . . .
VEGETARIAN

2 tablespoons flaxseed meal

1⅓ cups natural cashew or other nut butter

½ cup raw honey

2 teaspoons pure vanilla extract

½ cup cacao powder

Pinch of Himalayan pink salt

5 brown rice cakes, crushed into small pieces

Line an 8 by 8-inch pan with parchment paper.

In a medium bowl, combine the flaxseed meal, cashew butter, honey, vanilla, cacao powder, and salt. Mix thoroughly, then add the rice cake pieces and mix until the pieces are evenly coated.

Press the mixture into the pan, spreading it out evenly. Freeze 2 to 3 hours, until firm.

Slice into 9 squares to serve. Store leftovers in an airtight container in the refrigerator for up to 1 week.

# BERRY MEDLEY OAT CRUMBLE SQUARES

*B*reakfast or dessert? Your choice! When I make this recipe for guests, they assume it was a lot of work. It honestly takes me less than 10 minutes, and while I love fresh fruit, there are certain times of the year that I utilize a lot of organic frozen fruit. If you want to use fresh fruit, however, you could swap in any fruit that is currently in season. (Though apples, pears, and peaches would work the best!)

**SERVES 8**

Coconut oil, for the baking dish

1 cup frozen or fresh blueberries

¾ cup frozen or fresh raspberries

½ cup frozen or fresh blackberries

½ cup pure maple syrup or raw honey

2 teaspoons arrowroot or non-GMO cornstarch

¾ cup rolled oats or gluten-free oats

¾ cup almond flour

½ teaspoon baking powder

Pinch of sea salt

1 egg, lightly beaten

½ cup coconut oil, melted

2 teaspoons pure vanilla extract

⅓ cup sliced almonds

2 tablespoons pepitas

Preheat the oven to 350°F. Lightly coat an 8 by 8-inch baking dish with coconut oil.

In a small bowl, combine the blueberries, raspberries, blackberries, 2 tablespoons of the maple syrup, and the arrowroot. Set aside.

In a large bowl, combine the oats, almond flour, baking powder, and salt. Add the egg, the remaining maple syrup, the melted coconut oil, and vanilla and mix well.

Spread two-thirds of the oatmeal batter in the prepared baking dish. Spread the berry mixture evenly on top. Spread the remaining batter on top of the berries. Sprinkle the top of the crumb batter with the almonds and pepitas.

Bake until lightly golden brown, 25 to 30 minutes.

Cool completely before cutting into squares.

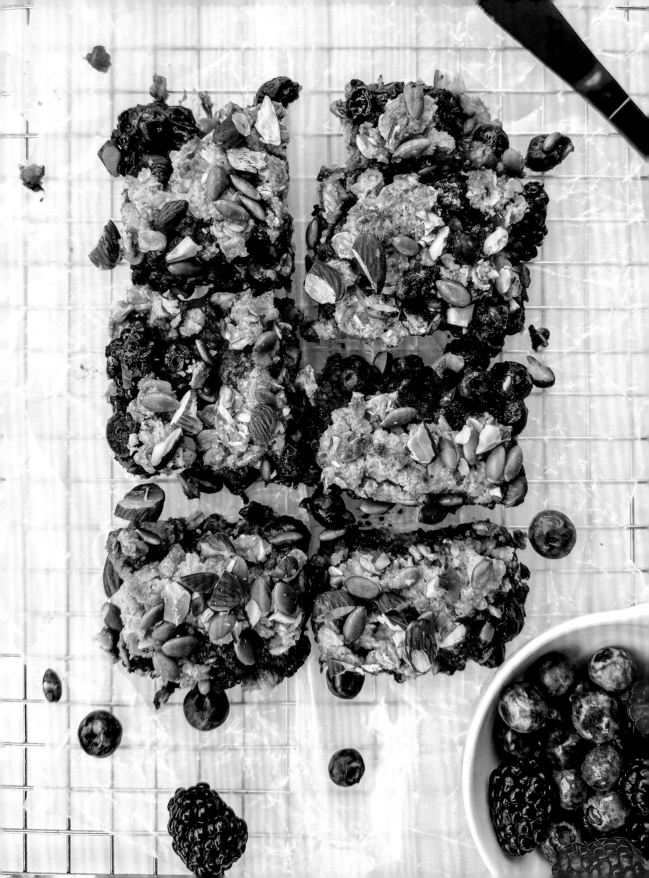

# CHEWY CHOCOLATE ENERGY BITES

As I was writing this chapter, I started thinking I might have a chocolate addiction. Eight out of fourteen dessert recipes have chocolate in them. That's more than half! But, so what if I do have a chocolate addiction? Chocolate has a fair amount of health benefits, as long as it's dark chocolate—the higher the cacao percentage, the better. Some studies have shown that the antioxidants found in cacao can actually improve cardiovascular health. The real question is, are the benefits emotional or physical, or both? I think both, and I think both are equally important. Eating chocolate makes me happy inside and out!

**MAKES 12 TO 16 BITES**

TO MAKE VEGETARIAN, USE VEGETARIAN PROTEIN POWDER INSTEAD OF COLLAGEN PEPTIDES.

1 cup rolled oats or gluten-free oats

⅓ cup flaxseed meal

¾ cup creamy natural nut butter

¼ cup raw honey

2 tablespoons unsweetened shredded coconut

1 scoop collagen peptides

½ cup mini dark chocolate chips

In a food processor, combine the oats, flaxseed meal, nut butter, honey, coconut, and collagen peptides. Pulse for 1 minute, or until the ingredients are mixed well and slightly sticky. Stir in the chocolate chips. With your hands, roll the mixture into 1- to 2-inch balls. Enjoy immediately or store in an airtight container in the refrigerator for up to 1 week.

# COOKIE DOUGH ENERGY BITES

*A*ny time we travel, whether it's for sports or for fun, or even if I'm sending my husband on a guys' trip, I pack these to go. They can serve as a meal in a pinch if you can't find the food you're looking for on the road, and they can be toted in a baggie rather than a container. You could even add some superfoods to them, like seeds or collagen peptides. If you're in the mood for cookies but short on baking time, this recipe will do the trick.

**MAKES 25 TO 30 ENERGY BITES**
. . . . . . . . . . . . . . . . . . . . . . .
VEGETARIAN

1¼ cups natural cashew or other nut/seed butter

½ cup raw honey

2 teaspoons pure vanilla extract

2 cups rolled oats or gluten-free oats

½ cup flaxseed meal

3 tablespoons unsweetened shredded coconut

½ teaspoon ground cinnamon

½ cup mini dark chocolate chips

Coconut oil (optional), melted

In a microwave-safe medium bowl, combine the cashew butter and honey and heat for 30 seconds. Stir to combine, then stir in the vanilla.

In a separate medium bowl, combine the oats, flaxseed meal, coconut, cinnamon, and chocolate chips. Add the cashew butter mixture to the dry mixture and stir well to combine. If the mixture is too dry, add melted coconut oil until all the ingredients are well incorporated.

Use a cookie scoop, a spoon, or your hands to portion the dough into 2-inch balls. Store the bites in the fridge or freezer.

## TIPS FOR FEEL-GOOD SLEEP

Our most important components of health—sleep, food, stress, exercise—are constantly working together and affecting how good or bad we feel. For a better night's sleep, every one of these components plays a part.

Cortisol is our stress hormone, and melatonin is our sleep hormone. They work together: When cortisol goes down, melatonin goes up and we start to feel sleepy. When cortisol goes up, melatonin goes down, and instead of feeling sleepy, we feel anxious and wound up. We've all been there! Here are some pointers for regulating cortisol and melatonin and for getting a better night's sleep.

- When you eat real food during the day, food that fits within the Feel-Good Way guidelines, you are taking in and using the nutrients you need to regulate your hormones and best manage all your other body systems—digestive, nervous, excretory, and more. All this supports good sleep. So, eat within the guidelines and drink plenty of water, and you'll be fueling yourself for better sleep.

- Stop eating for the day at least two hours before you go to bed. If your body is still digesting food, it's not getting or sending the message that it's time to wind down.

- Exercise helps alleviate stress, and the right amount of exercise uses your energy in a way that makes you feel ready for bed and a good night's sleep. Your movement can raise your cortisol level temporarily, which in turn means a reduced level later when you're ready to start winding down for the night. If your workouts are too intense, however, your cortisol levels could stay high for too long and interfere with your sleep. It's key to find that sweet spot of exercise without overdoing it. Including resistance training as part of your workouts is often especially helpful in regulating cortisol levels throughout the day and into the night.

- Breathwork and meditation also reduce cortisol levels and stress in general. See page 116 for one of my favorite breathing exercises.

- Ever been lying in bed and you can't quiet your mind? Keep a journal by your bed so you can sit up for a minute when needed and get those thoughts down on paper instead. Getting your worries on paper helps you cut off the continued angst running on repeat in your head. I find writing down what's bothering me helpful, even during the day when I feel overwhelmed, and especially at night.

- Avoid caffeine after noon. If you're exercising at the right intensity level and eating within the Feel-Good guidelines, you should have enough energy to wean yourself off the afternoon caffeine fix.

- Eliminate late-night alcohol.

- Create your own bedtime routine, such as reading, prayer, and/or journaling before you let your body and mind drift off for the night.

- If you're still having trouble sleeping and you feel like high stress and high cortisol are the leading causes, you may want to try a therapeutic cortisol manager supplement.

# CHEESECAKE BITES

*I*f you're a fan of cheesecake, I can't wait to hear what you think about these bites. As I've mentioned, in order to create a sustainable lifestyle, it's important to keep your favorites within reach. That doesn't mean you need to indulge daily in foods that aren't working for your whole body. But why not have it all when possible? Use foods that work for the whole body *and* feel like you're having an indulgence, without the negative effects.

**MAKES 12 BITES**

**VEGETARIAN**

**CRUST**

1 cup pitted dates

1 cup almond meal

1 tablespoon flaxseed meal

½ tablespoon grated orange zest

1 tablespoon coconut oil, melted

**CHEESECAKE**

One 8-ounce container nondairy cream cheese (such as Kite Hill)

1 cup canned full-fat coconut milk

¼ cup coconut oil

2 tablespoons pure maple syrup

2 tablespoons orange juice

Grated zest and juice of 1 lemon

1 scoop collagen peptides (optional)

¼ cup pomegranate seeds, for garnish

To make the crust: In a blender or food processor, combine the dates, almond meal, flaxseed meal, orange zest, and 1 tablespoon melted coconut oil. Blend in small pulses, until a sticky dough forms, adding 1 to 2 tablespoons water if needed for the desired consistency.

Line 12 cups of a muffin tin with cupcake liners or use silicone muffin cups. Place 1 tablespoon of the dough in the bottom of each cup. Press the dough down with your fingertips to make sure the dough is well packed. Place the muffin tin in the freezer to set for at least 15 minutes.

To make the cheesecake: In a blender or food processor, combine the cream cheese, coconut milk, coconut oil, maple syrup, orange juice, lemon zest, lemon juice, and collagen peptides (if using). Blend for 1 to 2 minutes, until smooth and creamy.

Divide the cream cheese mixture among the muffin cups, covering the crust. Sprinkle the pomegranate seeds on top of each cup, then place the muffin tin back in the freezer to set for at least 1 hour.

When ready to serve, remove the bites from the freezer and let them sit at room temperature for 5 to 10 minutes. Store bites in an airtight container in the freezer for 3 to 4 months.

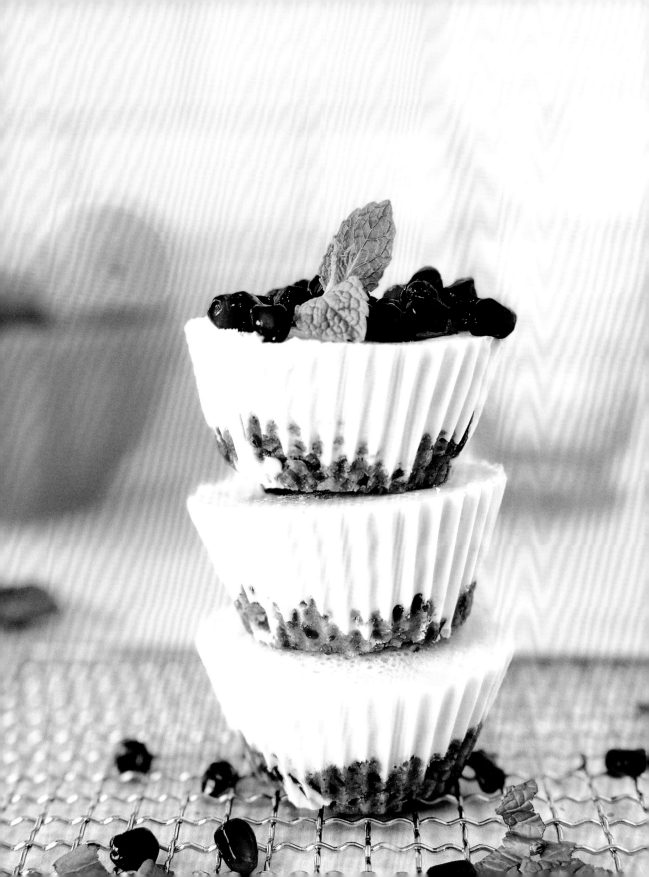

# MUG CAKE

Sometimes cravings come quickly, and if we don't act fast, it can turn ugly. Cravings aren't always a bad thing. Often they're a sign that our body is lacking minerals like magnesium and chromium. Other times they're just an indication of a hormone shift or unstable mood. The thing I've learned is, if you're using addictive foods like artificial flavors and sugar to sustain your cravings, then you'll need to eat more and more of them to satisfy your cravings. If you're eating real food, with fiber and nutrients, your cravings aren't as intense, and you only need a reasonable amount to satisfy them. This mug cake can be the quick fix you're looking for: quick to make and quick to enjoy!

## SERVES 1

Coconut oil cooking spray

1 egg, beaten

¼ cup rolled oats or gluten-free oats

2 tablespoons almond flour

¼ cup unsweetened nondairy milk

½ teaspoon pure vanilla extract

1 tablespoon flaxseed meal

1 teaspoon coconut oil, melted

### TOPPINGS

½ banana, sliced

Sprinkle of ground cinnamon

1 tablespoon chopped walnuts

1 teaspoon raw honey

Spritz a mug with coconut oil spray. Add the egg, oats, almond flour, milk, vanilla, flaxseed meal, and coconut oil. Mix until fully incorporated.

Cook in the microwave for 2 minutes to 2 minutes 30 seconds, or until cooked thoroughly. Add the toppings and enjoy.

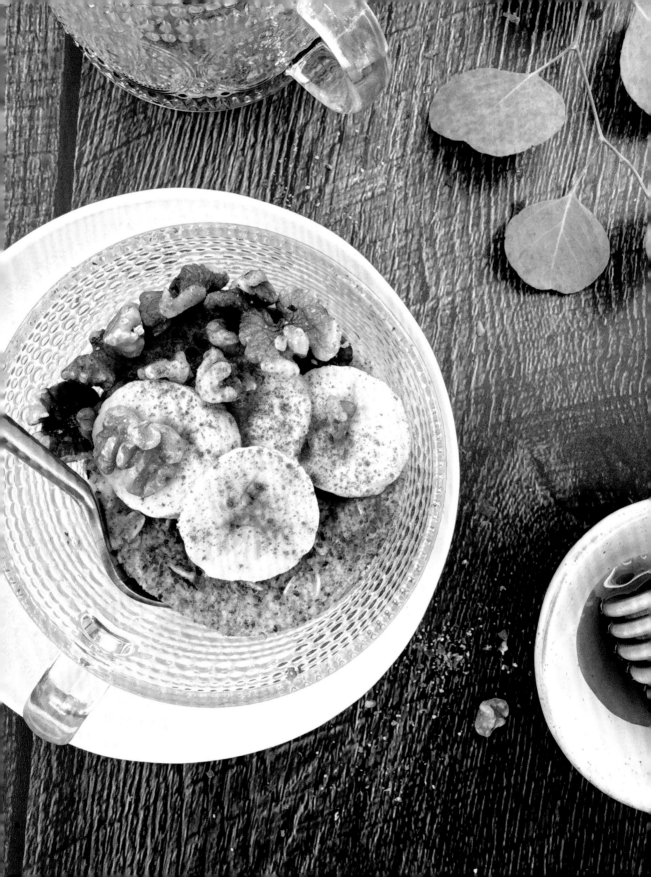

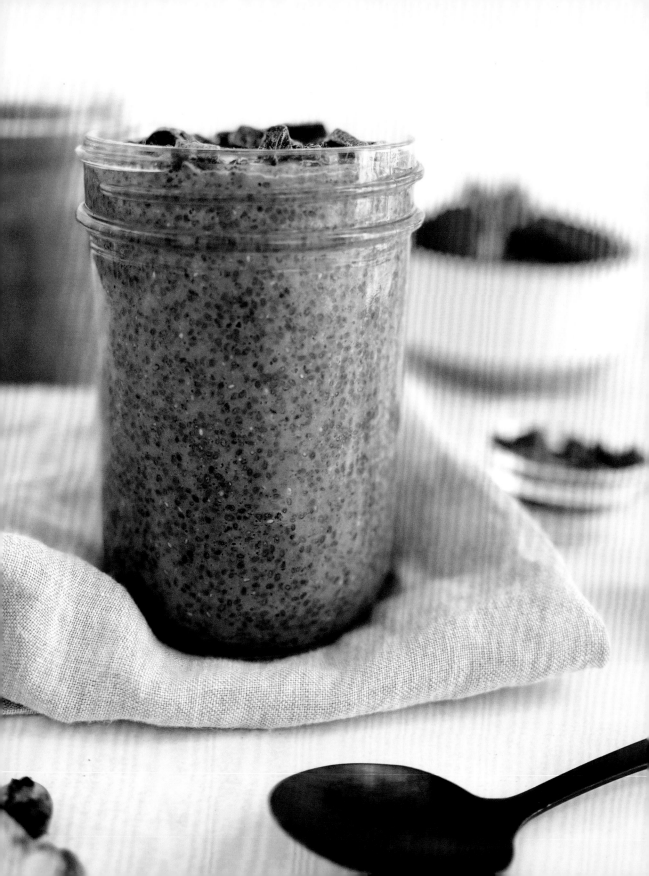

# CHIA PUDDING

*C*hia pudding is like regular pudding but pumped up with omega-3s and other health-optimizing foods. It's light and fluffy, due to the way chia seeds change when they come in contact with liquid. You may be surprised how sweetly satisfying the dates are in this recipe as well. It's an enjoyable option for when you're just starting to make changes into the Feel-Good philosophy or if you're already a Feel-Good expert. Chia pudding doesn't give you the sugar crash or guilt that more traditional, conventional puddings may.

**SERVES 2**

VEGETARIAN

1 cup unsweetened coconut or nut milk

4 tablespoons chia seeds

3 tablespoons natural almond or other nut/seed butter

2 tablespoons cacao powder

2 teaspoons maca powder

3 to 4 pitted dates, to taste

Dash of Himalayan pink salt

Cacao nibs (optional), for serving

Berries (optional), for serving

In a blender, combine the coconut milk, chia seeds, almond butter, cacao powder, maca powder, dates, and salt. Blend on medium for 5 minutes.

Divide the mixture between two 1-pint mason jars. Seal and refrigerate for 1 to 2 hours, or overnight.

If desired, serve topped with a sprinkle of cacao nibs and berries.

# SOUTHERN PEACH COBBLER

Nothing says summertime like cobbler. Where I grew up, blackberries grew wild and rampant. As a kid, it was fun to scavenge for them and see how many my brothers and sisters and I could pick. My aunt used to give us a large bowl and said if we could fill it, she would make us cobbler. It was a cake-like cobbler, but in the South, cobblers seem to be a little more crumbly, which I really love. This recipe is in the Southern style. I also realized over time that I much prefer peaches to berries in my cobbler. So I never let peach season pass without making this treat, but any fruit can be used.

**SERVES 6 TO 8**

- ¼ cup salted ghee or grass-fed butter
- 1½ cups finely ground almond flour
- ¼ cup arrowroot or tapioca starch
- ½ teaspoon baking powder
- ½ teaspoon sea salt
- Dash of ground nutmeg (optional)
- Dash of ground cinnamon (optional)
- ½ cup canned full-fat coconut milk
- ¼ cup plus 1 tablespoon pure maple syrup
- 1 egg
- ½ teaspoon pure vanilla extract
- 6 medium peaches, peeled and sliced
- Nondairy vanilla ice cream (such as Coconut Bliss or Nada Moo), for serving

Preheat the oven to 350°F. Place the ghee in the bottom of an 8 by 8-inch glass or ceramic baking dish. Put the dish in the oven while it's preheating for a few minutes to let the ghee melt. Use a silicone spatula to spread the melted ghee up the sides of the dish. Set aside.

In a medium bowl, whisk together the almond flour, arrowroot, baking powder, salt, nutmeg (if using), and cinnamon (if using). Add the coconut milk, maple syrup, egg, and vanilla. Whisk everything until well combined, but do not overmix.

Pour the batter into the prepared baking dish and smooth a little with the spatula. Layer the peaches on top of the batter, pressing them in slightly.

Bake until browned around the edges and on top, 42 to 47 minutes.

Let the cobbler cool for about 20 minutes before serving.

Serve with a scoop of ice cream.

# NICE CREAM

Wwe don't usually keep ice cream at home. I'm all for real ice cream, but I think everything is more enjoyable when there is an experience created around it, and some of my favorite childhood memories involve going out to get ice cream. Having said that, there are times when you're having ice cream cravings and it's not really time for a memorable experience. When that happens, nice cream it is!

SERVES 4
. . . . . . . . . . . . . . . . . . . . . .
TO MAKE VEGETARIAN,
USE VEGETARIAN PROTEIN
POWDER INSTEAD OF
COLLAGEN PEPTIDES.

1 frozen banana

2 teaspoons maple syrup
   or raw honey

½ teaspoon pure vanilla
   extract

2 tablespoons coconut
   cream

1 tablespoon natural
   cashew or other nut
   butter

½ scoop collagen peptides

Sprinkle of sea salt

In a blender or food processor, combine the banana, maple syrup, vanilla, coconut cream, cashew butter, collagen peptides, and salt. Blend to combine. Spread the mixture onto a sheet pan and freeze. After freezing for a couple of hours, scoop the nice cream using an ice cream scoop to serve.

# NICE CREAM SANDWICH

My girls have recently gotten into making nice cream sandwiches when they're having friends over. This nice cream sandwich, sure to impress even your healthiest foodie friends, tastes so good that you'll forget all the health benefits while you're enjoying it. To switch it up, you could always swap your favorite healthy ice cream for the nice cream, or you could alternate your favorite healthy cookies instead of using the Gluten-Free Chewy Chocolate Chunk Cookies. As always, feel free to be as creative as you'd like with these recipes.

**MAKES 1 SANDWICH**

· · · · · · · · · · · · · · · · · · · · · · ·

VEGETARIAN IF YOU USE A
FLAX/CHIA EGG (SEE PAGE 39)
IN THE COOKIES

⅓ cup Nice Cream (page 241)

2 Gluten-Free Chewy Chocolate Chunk Cookies (page 224)

Scoop nice cream onto a cookie, then place the second cookie on top to make a sandwich. Freeze the sandwich until set before serving.

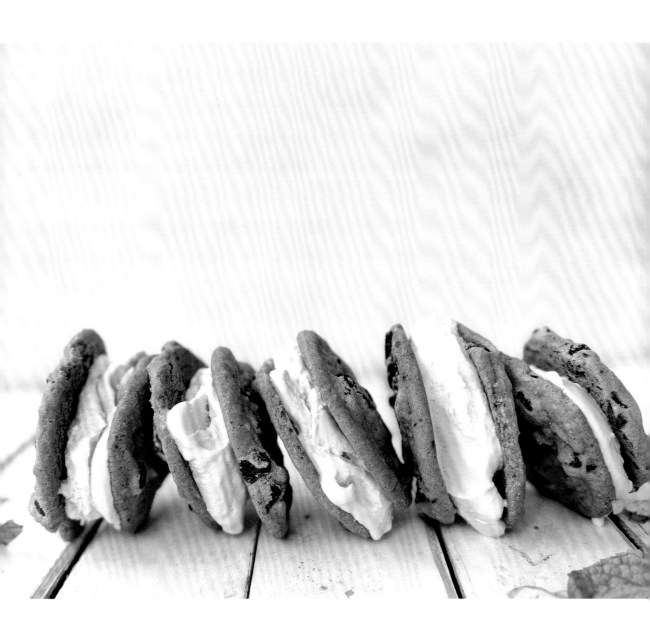

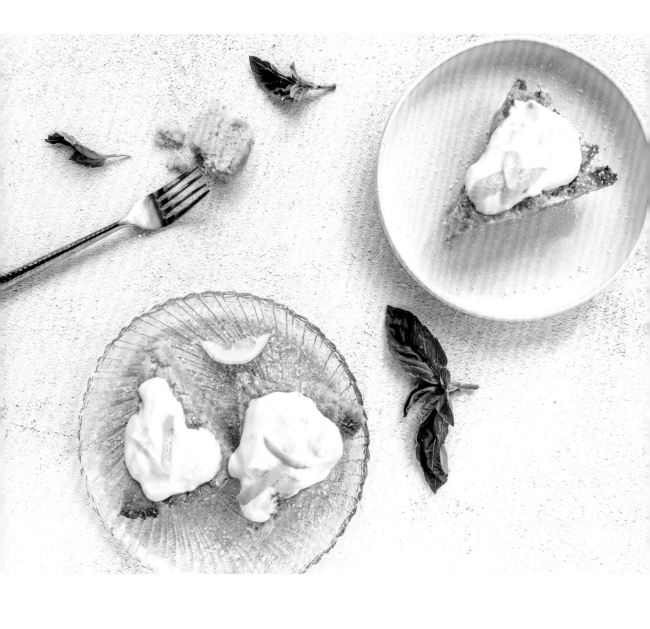

# LEMON CAKE

*M*y mom always said she hated any lemon dessert, so I never paid lemons much attention. When I got older and tried a lemon dessert on my own, well . . . it was a flavor explosion I'll never forget! I've been obsessed ever since. This lemon cake feels light and incredibly satisfying, particularly if you like the combination of slightly tart and slightly sweet as much as I do.

**SERVES 12**

2¼ cups almond flour

½ cup gluten-free flour

½ teaspoon baking soda

Dash of sea salt

3 eggs

½ cup pure maple syrup

⅓ cup grass-fed butter

2 tablespoons grated lemon zest

⅓ cup fresh lemon juice

1 teaspoon pure vanilla extract

**OPTIONAL GLAZE**

5 ounces full-fat plain Greek yogurt

2 tablespoons fresh lemon juice

2 tablespoons raw honey

2 tablespoons powdered sugar

Preheat the oven to 350°F. Line a 9 by 9-inch baking pan with parchment paper.

In a medium bowl, combine the almond flour, gluten-free flour, baking soda, and salt. In a large bowl, combine the eggs, maple syrup, butter, lemon zest, lemon juice, and vanilla. Whisk until well combined. One cup at a time, add the flour mixture to the wet mixture, stirring well. Pour the batter into the prepared pan.

Bake until a toothpick comes out clean, 25 to 30 minutes.

Let the cake cool completely in the pan.

If desired, make a glaze: In a small bowl, combine the yogurt, lemon juice, honey, and powdered sugar. Whisk well to combine. Drizzle the glaze over the cooled cake.

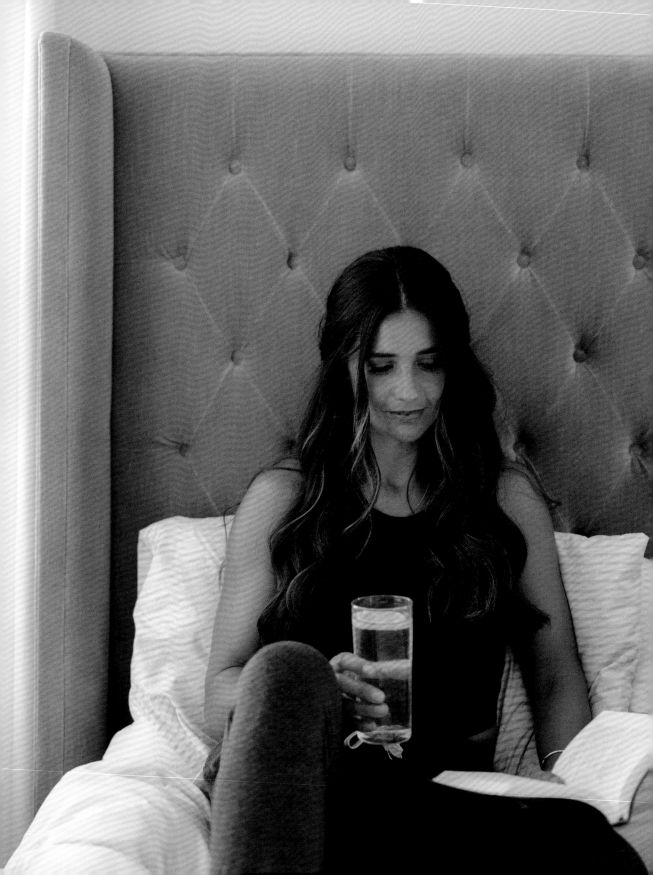

# END-OF-DAY PRAYER

***At the end*** of the day, we sometimes feel like we didn't get enough done, or we start to worry about the next day and what all we need to accomplish. That's why I find it important to pause at the end of the day to reflect, pray, breathe, and practice being thankful. I focus my prayer mostly on gratitude and any special intentions I have for the next day.

Bringing life back to gratitude is a very grounding practice, no matter where your faith walk stands. It has been shown to help reduce anxiety and relax our minds. For me, when I focus on what I'm truly grateful for and remember that I need for nothing, it resets my mind frame, calms me down, and brings me back to the present moment.

Because our family's life is pretty chaotic in the evenings, with our girls' activities and sports practices, I like to do this practice one-on-one with each kid. I love spending time as a family and sharing what we're grateful for, but it isn't always feasible for us. So, typically my husband and I do this with each of our kids separately, as they're getting ready for bed.

### God, we are thankful for . . .

List three different things you are thankful for as a family.

### God, I am thankful for . . .

Name one specific experience that happened to you personally today. Truthfully, it doesn't have to be good. It could just be a learning experience.

After spending time in gratitude, my husband and I always take time to pray over their sleep as well.

***Lord, in your name,*** I bless [their name]'s sleep to be restorative and healing. I bless their dreams to be comforting and peaceful, and I bless them to fall into their night of rest with relaxation and ease. I bless their minds to be calm, and I bless them to be protected in your coat of armor. We ask [any specific intentions over them now—a big test, big game, health issues, and so on]. We pray this in your name. Amen.

Later, as I lie down in bed, I close my eyes and ask the same over myself and my husband. I ask God to heal any loose ends or wounds in our marriage and bless us to grow in love and family unity. I bless peace over our home and then focus on what I am grateful for.

I wish I could say this is how I fall asleep every night! But after saying my prayers, if I can't drift off, I typically pick up whatever novel I'm into and fall asleep reading. I'm a chronic reader and would rather lose myself in a fun book than watch TV. Reading helps take my mind off my upcoming schedule or whatever items from my to-do list I didn't get to that day. Instead, I'm focusing on solving the mystery of whatever crime, suspense, or psychological thriller I'm reading. Reading helps me be in the present moment. For some reason, TV doesn't do that for me.

Relaxation, however you find it, is in itself a gift from God. I'm not sure my younger self fully appreciated it, but now I think of it as yet another blessing I'm so thankful for. Prayer and rest go well together. Prayer helps us to surrender, to take a load off, to focus our intentions without the feeling of total control. It helps us reframe our minds and ultimately gain more peace and comfort, which puts us in a restful state.

After a day of Feel-Good food, finding the present moment in prayer or breathwork, and nourishing your body and mind, you will hopefully also feel very proud of yourself. Going to bed in a state of gratitude and accomplishment is a great way to invite deep, productive sleep and nurture yourself on an even deeper level. You can feel overwhelmed when feeling good has slipped away, but always remember, you're just one meal away from resetting and getting yourself back on the right track. I often say, little by little, a little becomes a lot.

# PARTING BLESSING

***I believe we're*** all meant to feel good. Yes, all of us will experience suffering to different degrees, but I truly believe all of us were meant for more. Feeling good is a gift that we should never take for granted.

For some reason, it's easier to notice when we don't feel good than it is to appreciate when we do. When you're not feeling great, you say it out loud, you tell other people, you spend time thinking about it. When we wake up and we feel good, we need to give that experience the same attention. Tell yourself, *Wow, I feel good today.* Tell other people, *I feel really good today,* and see what they say. Let's not let good days pass without acknowledging them.

We all know the phrase "one day at a time," but I want to remind you that when we're talking about the gift of feeling good, it's one *meal* at a time. Each meal is an opportunity to fuel your body the best way possible. It's an opportunity to trust your intuition. It's an opportunity to make a positive difference in how you feel. One meal at a time.

You don't have to wait for a Monday or the first of the month or a new year: All you need is the next meal. This isn't about being perfect, it's about giving yourself a chance to feel your best. One thing I can promise you is that the Feel-Good Way will lead to a Feel-Good Life. I pray this becomes a reality for you, no matter how much time it takes. You are worth it.

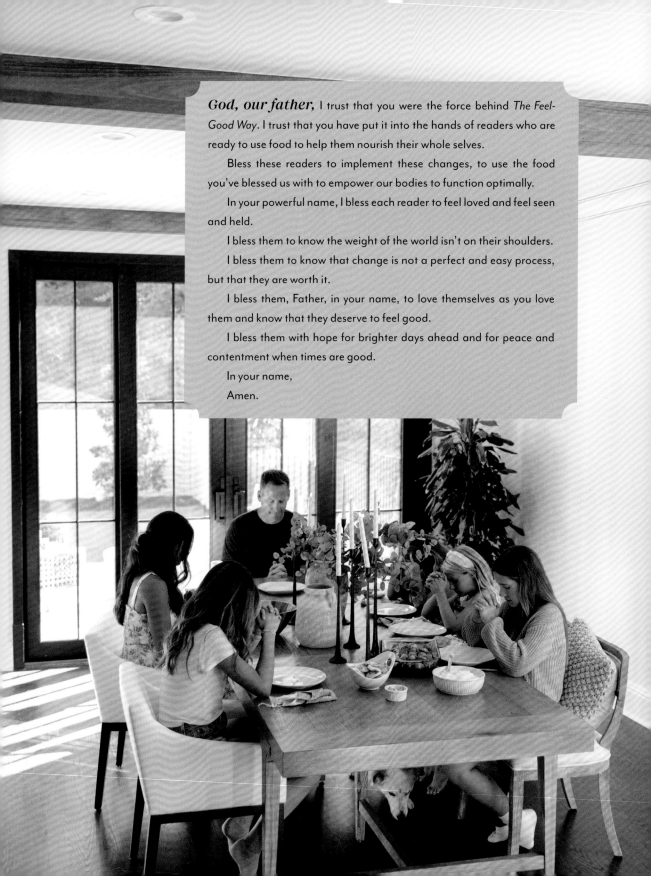

*God, our father,* I trust that you were the force behind *The Feel-Good Way*. I trust that you have put it into the hands of readers who are ready to use food to help them nourish their whole selves.

Bless these readers to implement these changes, to use the food you've blessed us with to empower our bodies to function optimally.

In your powerful name, I bless each reader to feel loved and feel seen and held.

I bless them to know the weight of the world isn't on their shoulders.

I bless them to know that change is not a perfect and easy process, but that they are worth it.

I bless them, Father, in your name, to love themselves as you love them and know that they deserve to feel good.

I bless them with hope for brighter days ahead and for peace and contentment when times are good.

In your name,

Amen.

# ACKNOWLEDGMENTS

This book couldn't have happened without the dream team. My editor, Derek, understood the vision and the mission, and I couldn't be more thankful our visions completely aligned. My agent, Amy, not only believed in me but also believes in the greater need for sustainable health. I'm thankful for this journey with Amy and all the hard work it took to get us to this point. My collaborative writer, Bessie, is an absolute visionary and so calming. It's like she knows what I teach even better than I do. I couldn't be more thankful to have a collaborative writer who not only grasped the concepts but even implemented them in her own life. I'm so thankful to God for the journey that this book took to transpire! I'm also thankful for the entire Convergent team who has blessed this opportunity with their skills. Thank you, Tina Constable, Campbell Wharton, Jessalyn Foggy, Elizabeth Groening, Steve Boriack, Alisse Goldsmith-Wissman, Ashley Shoemaker, Elizabeth Rendfleisch, Jessie Bright, and Abby Duval.

Thank you, Carrie, for blessing me with your honest foreword for this book. You've helped me change so many lives for the better, and I'm eternally grateful for that!

I'm grateful for my incredibly talented photographer, Kim. She crushed it, making food dreams come true with these amazing photos. She has also developed recipes for CCN, for which I'm also so thankful. Kim, keep inspiring the world with your gifts! Thanks also to Anjelica, who did an amazing job with the lifestyle photography for this book.

I couldn't have done this without my team at Cara Clark Nutrition. Ashlee, you're my right hand and the left brain to my right brain—or the other way around. You help me stay on task and quickly deliver bits and pieces along the way. I literally couldn't carry on with my workload without you. Allison, you're my dedicated recipe developer and top-notch nutritionist at CCN. You're ingrained in every aspect of all the work I put out. Thank you, Ashlee and Allison! Thank you, Mia, my dedicated partner in marketing, and Abbey, my dedicated PR and all-things-social gal. Thanks also to the rest of the CCN team: Audrey, Amelia, and Nellie. God really knew what he was doing by putting this force together for good!

Last but not least, I'm beyond grateful for my personal taste-testing team, my family: my husband of sixteen years, our four daughters, and our leftover queen, Aspen the dog. My girls inspire every ounce of work I do. They are my greatest teacher, motivator, and life-giving inspiration. If it weren't for their support and patience, we couldn't have finished this.

Thank you to my CCN members who inspire me to offer more amazing recipes to help nourish and heal and sustain you all. This is all for nothing, if not for y'all!

Overall, I'm blessed and certainly couldn't have accomplished this alone! I'm so thankful for the people God places in my path for the greater good! Many blessings to you, my readers. I pray this book changes your life!

# INDEX

# ABOUT THE AUTHOR

Cara Clark is an integrative nutritionist and wellness educator, certified in sports and clinical nutrition. As the founder of Cara Clark Nutrition, she has worked with thousands of clients, including celebrities, Olympic athletes, and NBA and MLB draft prospects, to help them feel better in their bodies. She is the primary nutritionist for the fitness app and online community fit52 and contributed to the book *Find Your Path: Honor Your Body, Fuel Your Soul, and Get Strong with the Fit52 Life* by Carrie Underwood. Clark also co-authored *The Wellness Remodel: A Guide to Rebooting How You Eat, Move, and Feed Your Soul*. Clark lives in Nashville, Tennessee, with her husband and their four girls.